The Tobacco Atlas

"When one has a thorough knowledge of both the enemy and oneself, victory is assured. When one has a thorough knowledge of both heaven and earth, victory will be complete."

— General Sun Tzu
The Art of War: A Treatise on Chinese Military Science
c. 500 B.C.

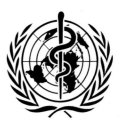

Publications of the World Health Organization
can be obtained from:

Marketing and Dissemination
World Health Organization
20 Avenue Appia
1211 Geneva 27
Switzerland
tel: +41 22 791 2476
fax: +41 22 791 4857
email: bookorders@who.int

Requests for permission to reproduce or
translate WHO publications – whether for sale
or for noncommercial distribution – should
be addressed to:

Publications
address as above
fax: +41 22 791 4806
email: permissions@who.int

The designations employed and the presentation of
the material in this publication do not imply the
expression of any opinion whatsoever on the part
of the World Health Organization concerning the
legal status of any country, territory, city or area or
of its authorities, or concerning the delimitation of
its frontiers or boundaries. Dotted lines on maps
represent approximate border lines for which there
may not yet be full agreement.

The mention of specific companies or of certain
manufacturers' products does not imply that they
are endorsed or recommended by the World
Health Organization in preference to others of a
similar nature that are not mentioned. Errors and
omissions excepted, the names of proprietary
products are distinguished by initial capital letters.

The World Health Organization does not
warrant that the information contained in this
publication is complete and correct and shall not
be liable for any damages incurred as a result of its
use.

The authors alone are responsible for the views
expressed in this publication.

The Tobacco Atlas

Dr Judith Mackay
and Dr Michael Eriksen

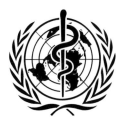

The Tobacco Atlas © World Health Organization 2002

First published 2002
10 9 8 7 6 5 4 3 2 1

ISBN 92 4156 209 9

Produced for the World Health Organization by
Myriad Editions Limited
6–7 Old Steine, Brighton BN1 1EJ, UK
http://www.MyriadEditions.com

Edited and co-ordinated for Myriad Editions by
Paul Jeremy and Candida Lacey
Design and graphics by Paul Jeremy
and Corinne Pearlman
Maps created by Isabelle Lewis

Printed and bound in Hong Kong
Produced by Phoenix Offset Limited
under the supervision of Bob Cassels,
The Hanway Press, London

CONTENTS

FOREWORD

A message from

**Dr Gro Harlem Bruntland
Director-General
World Health Organization**

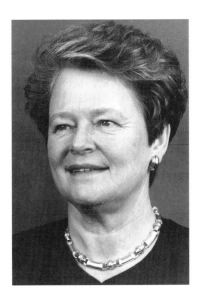

"More people smoke today than at any other time in human history. One person dies every ten seconds due to smoking-related diseases.

Research evidence in the past five years shows a bleaker picture of the health danger of smoking than previously realised. Tobacco is the biggest killer, much bigger in dimension than all other forms of pollution.

Children are the most vulnerable. Habits start in youth. The tobacco industry knows it and acts accordingly. This is a medical challenge, but also a cultural challenge. Let us all speak out: tobacco is a killer. It should not be advertised, subsidised or glamourised.

Adolescents should not be allowed to mortgage their lives to the seductive advertisements of the industry. Girls and women are being targeted all over the world by expensive and seductive tobacco advertising images of freedom, emancipation, slimness, glamour and wealth. Tobacco companies should be accountable for the harm caused by tobacco use.

The day I took office I launched the Tobacco Free Initiative (TFI) to spearhead the struggle to reverse the worsening trends in health caused by tobacco and to add momentum to a critical public health struggle. The initiative aims at heightening global awareness of the need to address tobacco consumption. It also seeks to build new partnerships and strengthen existing partnerships for action against tobacco; to commission policy research to fill gaps; and, to accelerate national and global policy to implement strategies.

The way it works illustrates the way we wish WHO to work in the future making the most of our own resources and knowledge and drawing heavily on the knowledge and experience of others.

Our goals are to:
• build "a vibrant alliance" between WHO, UNICEF, the World Bank, and "partnerships with a purpose" with non governmental organisations, the private sector, academic/research institutions and donors.

• try to get more people to work on and support tobacco control activities and ensure that more resources are committed to tobacco research, policy and control.

• develop the Framework Convention on Tobacco Control (FCTC), the world's first public health treaty. The treaty will only be effective if it works in conjunction with, and builds upon, sound domestic interventions.

The good news is that the epidemic does not have to continue this way. There is a political solution to tobacco – a solution routed through ministries of finance and agriculture as well as health and education.

We know that tobacco control measures can lead to a reduction in smoking as witnessed among some member states. WHO, the World Bank and public health experts have identified a combination of the following as having a measurable and sustained impact on tobacco use:
• increased excise taxes;
• bans on tobacco advertising, sponsorship and

marketing;
- controls on smoking in public places and workplaces;
- expanded access to effective means of quitting;
- tough counteradvertising;
- tight controls on smuggling.

These must all be implemented if the predicted expansion of the epidemic as outlined in this atlas is to be prevented.

The picture is far from bleak. Globally, we have seen a sea change over the past few years. A groundswell of local, national and global actions is moving the public health agenda ahead.

DR GRO HARLEM BRUNTLAND
Geneva
June 2002

PREFACE

This book is intended for anyone concerned with personal or political health, governance, politics, economics, big business, corporate behaviour, smuggling, tax, religion, internet, allocation of resources, human development and the future.

The atlas maps the history, current situation and some predictions for the future of the tobacco epidemic up to the year 2050.

It illustrates how tobacco is not just a simple health issue, but involves economics, big business, politics, trade and crimes such as smuggling, litigation and deceit.

The atlas also shows the importance of a multifaceted approach to reducing the epidemic – by WHO, other UN agencies, NGOs, the private sector and, in fact, the whole of civil society.

The publication of this atlas marks a critical time in the epidemic. We stand at a crossroads, with the future in our hands. We can choose to stand aside; or to take weak and ineffective measures; or to implement robust and enduring measures to protect the health and wealth of nations.

JUDITH MACKAY, Hong Kong
MICHAEL ERIKSEN, Geneva
June 2002

ACKNOWLEDGEMENTS

We would like to thank the Centers for Disease Control and Prevention (CDC), USA, for providing financial support for this atlas.

Many people have helped in the preparation of this atlas. Firstly our thanks to all those at the World Health Organization:

Headquarters, Geneva:

Joyce Bleeker, Noncommunicable Disease Prevention and Health Promotion (NPH), Noncommunicable Diseases and Mental Health Cluster (NMH);

Douglas Bettcher, Tobacco Free Initiative (TFI), Noncommunicable Diseases and Mental Health Cluster (NMH);

David Bramley, Health Information Management and Dissemination (IMD), Evidence and Information for Policy Cluster (EIP);

Gian Luca Burci, Office of the Legal Counsel (LEG);

Vera Luiza da Costa e Silva, Tobacco Free Initiative (TFI), Noncommunicable Diseases and Mental Health Cluster (NMH);

Emmanuel Guindon, Tobacco Free Initiative (TFI) Noncommunicable Diseases and Mental Health Cluster (NMH);

Ewa Carlsson Höpperger, Office of the Legal Counsel (LEG);

Prabhat Jha, Commission on Macroeconomics and Health (CMH), Evidence and Information for Policy Cluster (EIP);

Alan Lopez, Evidence and Information for Policy Cluster (EIP);

Garrett Mehl, Noncommunicable Disease Prevention and Health Promotion (NPH), Noncommunicable Diseases and Mental Health Cluster (NMH);

Diana Munoru, Noncommunicable Disease Prevention and Health Promotion (NPH), Noncommunicable Diseases and Mental Health Cluster (NMH);

El Atifi Mustapha, Tobacco Free Initiative (TFI), Noncommunicable Diseases and Mental Health Cluster (NMH);

Pekka Puska, Noncommunicable Disease Prevention and Health Promotion (NPH), Noncommunicable Diseases and Mental Health Cluster (NMH);

Leanne Riley, Noncommunicable Disease Prevention and Health Promotion (NPH), Noncommunicable Diseases and Mental Health Cluster (NMH);

Paula Soper, Tobacco Free Initiative (TFI), Noncommunicable Diseases and Mental Health Cluster (NMH);

Derek Yach, Noncommunicable Diseases and Mental Health Cluster (NMH).

Regional offices:

Karen Klimowski, Charles Maringo, AFRO;
Fatimah M S El Awa, EMRO;
Patsy Harrington, Haik Nikogosian, Ionela Petrea, EURO;
Heather Selin, Armando Peruga, PAHO;
Martha Osei, SEARO;
Harley Stanton, WPRO.

For their advice on particular maps and subjects, we would like to thank the following:

2. Types of Tobacco Use
Samira Asma, CDC, USA; Prakash Gupta, Tata Institute of Fundamental Research, India;

3. Male Smoking and 4. Female Smoking
Marlo Corrao, American Cancer Society, USA; Amanda Sandford, ASH UK;

5. Youth
GYTS Coordinators; Wick Warren, CDC, USA;

6. Cigarette Consumption
Tom Capehart, Economic Research Service, USDA; Prakash Gupta, Tata Institute of Fundamental Research, India;

7. Health Risks
Gary Giovino, Roswell Park Cancer Institute, USA; Corinne Pearlman, Comic Company, UK; Jonathan Samet, Johns Hopkins Institute for Global Tobacco Control, USA; Stan Shatenstein, Communications consultant, Canada;

8. Passive Smoking
Clive Bates, ASH UK; Corinne Pearlman, Comic Company, UK; Jonathan Samet, Johns Hopkins Institute for Global Tobacco Control, USA; Wick Warren, CDC, USA;

9. Deaths
Majid Ezzati, Resources for the Future, USA;

11. Costs to the Smoker
Luk Joossens, Belgium; Kenneth E Warner, University of Michigan, USA; Anna White, Partnership Programme, Essential Action's Taking on Tobacco campaign; Ayda A. Yurekli, The World Bank;

12. Growing Tobacco and **15. Tobacco Trade**
Tom Capehart, USDA;

14. Tobacco Companies
Gene Borio, New York City, USA;

16. Tobacco Smuggling
Campaign for Tobacco Free Kids, USA; Luk Joossens, Belgium; Eric LeGresley, Tobacco Control Consultant, Ottawa, Canada;

18. Internet Sales
Chris Banthin, NorthEastern University, Boston, USA; Greg Connolly, Mass Dept of Public Health, USA; Kurt M. Ribisl, University of North Carolina at Chapel Hill, USA; Kenneth Warner, University of Michigan, USA;

19. Politics
Sibylle Fleitmann, European Network for Smoking Prevention, Belgium; Anne Landman, Doc-Alert, Colorado, USA;

21. Tobacco Industry Documents
Lisa Bero, University of California, San Francisco, USA; Anne Landman, Colorado, USA; Jonathan Liberman, VicHealth Centre for Tobacco Control, Australia;

22. Research
Linda Waverly Brigden, IDRC, Ottawa, Canada; Sibylle Fleitmann, European Network for Smoking Prevention, Belgium; Rowena Jacobs, University of York, UK; Rosemary Kennedy, IDRC, Ottawa, Canada; Gerald Keusch, Fogarty International Center, NIH, USA; Aron Primack, Fogarty International Center, NIH, USA; Anthony So, Rockefeller, NYC, USA; Jacob Sweiry, Wellcome Trust, London, UK;

23. Tobacco Control Organisations
Sibylle Fleitmann, European Network for Smoking Prevention, Belgium; Belinda Hughes, Framework Convention Alliance, Australia; Ruben Israel, GLOBALink, International Union Against Cancer (UICC); Yussuf Saloojee, INGCAT, South Africa; David Simpson, International Agency on Tobacco and Health, UK;

24. Smoke-free Areas
Melanie Wakefield, Anti-Cancer Council of Victoria, Australia;

27. Health Education
Patrick Sandstrom, Quit & Win, Finland; Eeva Riitta Vartiainen, Quit & Win, Finland;

28. Quitting
Marlo Corrao, American Cancer Society, USA; GlaxoSmithKline; David Graham, World Self Medication Industry; Pharmacia; Jerry Reinstein, World Self Medication Industry; Pharmacia;

29. Price Policy
Gene Borio, NYC, USA; Frank Chaloupka, University of Illinois, USA; Anne Jones, ASH, Australia; Amanda Sandford, ASH UK; Michele Scollo, VicHealth Centre for Tobacco Control, Australia; Joy Townsend, London School of Hygiene and Tropical Medicine, University of London, UK.

For their general contributions, we would like to thank Kjell Bjartveit, John Crofton, Nigel Gray, Ruth Roemer, Michael Pertschuk and Weng Xinzhi; and, especially, John Mackay.

For their creative and editorial expertise, diverse talents, and individual as well as collective contributions, we would like to thank the team at Myriad Editions: Candida Lacey, Paul Jeremy, Isabelle Lewis and Corinne Pearlman.

Finally, we want to thank our respective families for their support during the preparation of this atlas.

PHOTO CREDITS

front cover:
Boy smoking, Seychelles
Credit: Harry Anenden © WHO

back cover:
Boy in the road selling packs to drivers and
passengers, Philippines
Credit: Daniel Tan

Woman tobacco worker, Vietnam
Credit: Judith Mackay

Men smoking water pipes, Saudi Arabia
Photo: Garrett Mehl

Part 1 **Prevalence and Health**
Man and child smoking, China
Credit: Carol Betson

Part 2 **The Cost of Tobacco**
Tobacco leaves, Thailand
Credit: Judith Mackay

Part 3 **The Tobacco Trade**
Woman tagging tobacco, tobacco factory,
Virginia, USA
Credit: Ken Hammond © USDA

Part 4 **Promotion**
Boy in the road selling packs to drivers and
passengers, Philippines
Credit: Daniel Tan

Part 5 **Taking Action**
"Smoking is Ugly" poster,
created by Christy Turlington and reprinted
courtesy of the Centers for Disease Control and
Prevention (CDC)

Part 6 **World Tables**
Old Man, Sri Lanka
Credit: Garrett Mehl

ABOUT THE AUTHORS

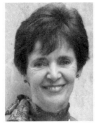

Dr Judith Mackay is a medical doctor and Senior Policy Advisor to the World Health Organization. She is based in Hong Kong where she is the Director of the Asian Consultancy on Tobacco Control. After an early career as a hospital physician, she became a health advocate. She is a Fellow of the Royal Colleges of Physicians of Edinburgh and London and the Hong Kong Academy of Medicine and author of *The State of Health Atlas* and *The Penguin Atlas of Human Sexual Behavior*. Dr Mackay has received many international awards including the WHO Commemorative Medal, the Fries Prize for Improving Health, the Luther Terry Award for Outstanding Individual Leadership, the International Partnering for World Health Award, and the Founding International Achievement Award from the Asia Pacific Association for the Control of Tobacco.

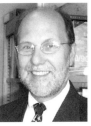

Dr Michael Eriksen is former Director of the U.S. Office on Smoking and Health and is currently a Distinguished Consultant at the Centers for Disease Control and Prevention in Atlanta. Since 2000, Dr. Eriksen has served as an Advisor to the World Health Organization in Geneva. He is a recipient of the WHO Commemorative Medal. He is a Past President and Distinguished Fellow of the Society for Public Health Education and is a thirty-year member of the American Public Health Association.

The History of Tobacco

"In ancient times, when the land was barren and the people were starving, the Great Spirit sent forth a woman to save humanity. As she travelled over the world everywhere her right hand touched the soil, there grew potatoes. And everywhere her left hand touched the soil, there grew corn. And in the place where she had sat, there grew tobacco." Huron Indian myth

"The Spaniards upon their journey met with great multitudes of people, men and women with firebrands in their hands and herbs to smoke after their custom."
Christopher Columbus' journal,
6 November 1492

"Smoking is a custom loathsome to the eye, hateful to the nose, harmful to the brain, dangerous to the lungs, and in the black, stinking fume thereof nearest resembling the horrible Stygian smoke of the pit that is bottomless."
James I of England
A Counterblaste to Tobacco 1604

"I say, if you can't send money, send tobacco."
first US President George Washington's request to help finance the American Civil War, 1776

Within 150 years of Columbus's finding "strange leaves" in the New World, tobacco was being used around the globe. Its rapid spread and widespread acceptance characterise the addiction to the plant *Nicotina tobacum*. Only the mode of delivery has changed. In the 18th century, snuff held sway; the 19th century was the age of the cigar; the 20th century saw the rise of the manufactured cigarette, and with it a greatly increased number of smokers. At the beginning of the 21st century about one third of adults in the world, including increasing numbers of women, used tobacco.

Despite thousands of studies showing that tobacco in all its forms kills its users, and smoking cigarettes kills non-users, people continue to smoke, and deaths from tobacco use continue to increase.

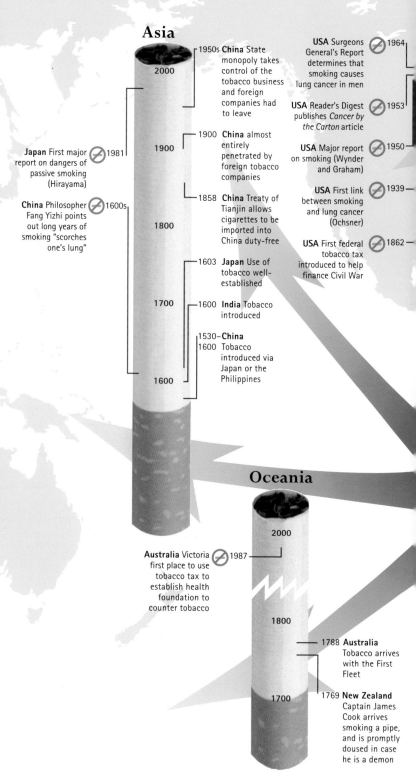

Asia

1950s **China** State monopoly takes control of the tobacco business and foreign companies had to leave

1900 **China** almost entirely penetrated by foreign tobacco companies

1858 **China** Treaty of Tianjin allows cigarettes to be imported into China duty-free

1603 **Japan** Use of tobacco well-established

1600 **India** Tobacco introduced

1530–1600 **China** Tobacco introduced via Japan or the Philippines

Japan First major report on dangers of passive smoking (Hirayama) — 1981

China Philosopher Fang Yizhi points out long years of smoking "scorches one's lung" — 1600s

USA Surgeons General's Report determines that smoking causes lung cancer in men — 1964

USA Reader's Digest publishes *Cancer by the Carton* article — 1953

USA Major report on smoking (Wynder and Graham) — 1950

USA First link between smoking and lung cancer (Ochsner) — 1939

USA First federal tobacco tax introduced to help finance Civil War — 1862

Oceania

Australia Victoria first place to use tobacco tax to establish health foundation to counter tobacco — 1987

1788 **Australia** Tobacco arrives with the First Fleet

1769 **New Zealand** Captain James Cook arrives smoking a pipe, and is promptly doused in case he is a demon

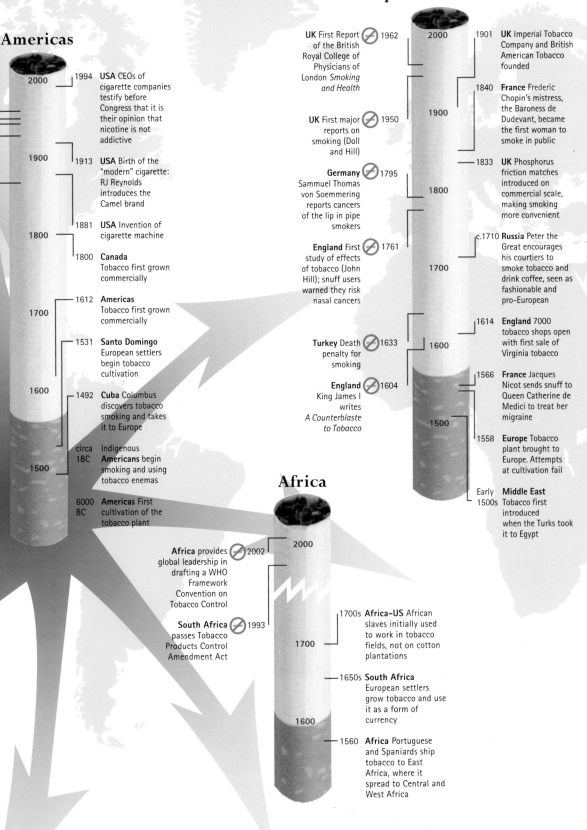

Americas

2000

- **1994 USA** CEOs of cigarette companies testify before Congress that it is their opinion that nicotine is not addictive

1900

- **1913 USA** Birth of the "modern" cigarette: RJ Reynolds introduces the Camel brand

1800

- **1881 USA** Invention of cigarette machine
- **1800 Canada** Tobacco first grown commercially

1700

- **1612 Americas** Tobacco first grown commercially
- **1531 Santo Domingo** European settlers begin tobacco cultivation

1600

- **1492 Cuba** Columbus discovers tobacco smoking and takes it to Europe
- **circa 1BC Indigenous Americans** begin smoking and using tobacco enemas

1500

- **6000 BC Americas** First cultivation of the tobacco plant

Europe and Middle East

2000

- **UK** First Report of the British Royal College of Physicians of London *Smoking and Health* — 1962
- **UK** First major reports on smoking (Doll and Hill) — 1950

1900

- **1901 UK** Imperial Tobacco Company and British American Tobacco founded
- **1840 France** Frederic Chopin's mistress, the Baroness de Dudevant, became the first woman to smoke in public
- **1833 UK** Phosphorus friction matches introduced on commercial scale, making smoking more convenient

1800

- **Germany** Sammuel Thomas von Soemmering reports cancers of the lip in pipe smokers — 1795
- **England** First study of effects of tobacco (John Hill); snuff users warned they risk nasal cancers — 1761

1700

- **c.1710 Russia** Peter the Great encourages his courtiers to smoke tobacco and drink coffee, seen as fashionable and pro-European
- **1614 England** 7000 tobacco shops open with first sale of Virginia tobacco

1600

- **Turkey** Death penalty for smoking — 1633
- **England** King James I writes *A Counterblaste to Tobacco* — 1604
- **1566 France** Jacques Nicot sends snuff to Queen Catherine de Medici to treat her migraine

1500

- **1558 Europe** Tobacco plant brought to Europe. Attempts at cultivation fail
- **Early 1500s Middle East** Tobacco first introduced when the Turks took it to Egypt

Africa

2000

- **Africa** provides global leadership in drafting a WHO Framework Convention on Tobacco Control — 2002
- **South Africa** passes Tobacco Products Control Amendment Act — 1993

1700

- **1700s Africa–US** African slaves initially used to work in tobacco fields, not on cotton plantations
- **1650s South Africa** European settlers grow tobacco and use it as a form of currency

1600

- **1560 Africa** Portuguese and Spaniards ship tobacco to East Africa, where it spread to Central and West Africa

19

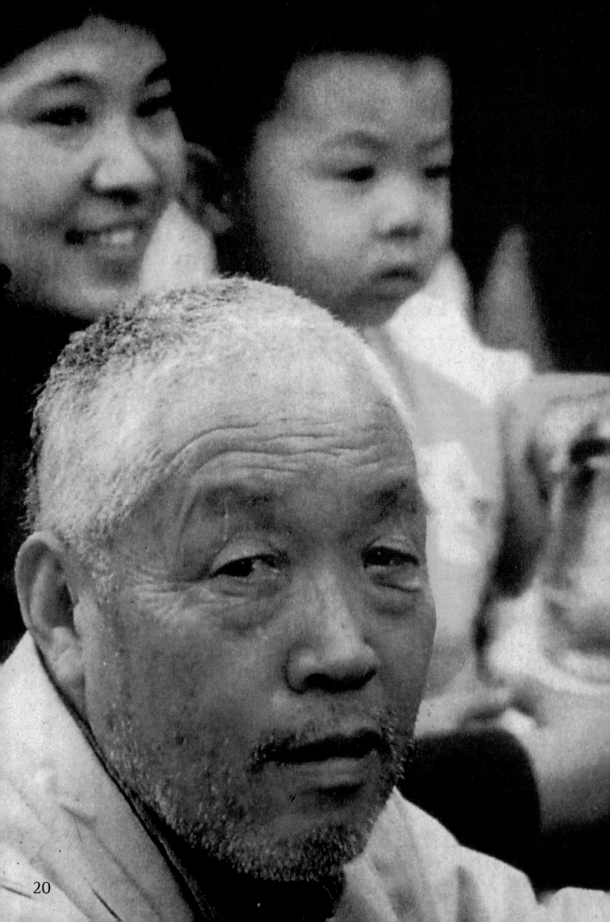

PART 1

PREVALENCE AND HEALTH

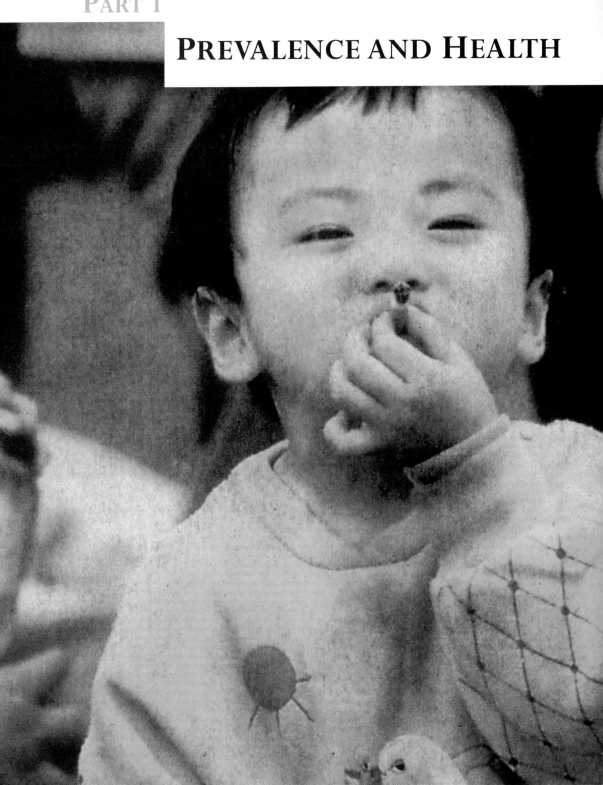

"... tobacco is the only legally available consumer product which kills people when it is entirely used as intended."

The Oxford Medical Companion, 1994

2 | Types of Tobacco Use

Smoking tobacco

Manufactured cigarettes consist of shredded or reconstituted tobacco processed with hundreds of chemicals. Often with a filter, they are manufactured by a machine, and are the predominant form of tobacco used worldwide.

Bidis consist of a small amount of tobacco, hand-wrapped in dried temburni leaf and tied with string. Despite their small size, their tar and carbon monoxide deliveries can be higher than manufactured cigarettes because of the need to puff harder to keep bidis lit.

Cigars are made of air-cured and fermented tobaccos with a tobacco wrapper, and come in many shapes and sizes, from cigarette-sized cigarillos, double coronas, cheroots, stumpen, chuttas and dhumtis. In reverse chutta and dhumti smoking, the ignited end of the cigar is placed inside the mouth. There was a revival of cigar smoking at the end of the 20th century, among both men and women.

Kreteks are clove-flavoured cigarettes. They contain a wide range of exotic flavourings and eugenol, which has an anaesthetising effect, allowing for deeper smoke inhalation.

Pipes are made of briar, slate, clay or other substance – tobacco is placed in the bowl and inhaled through the stem, sometimes through water.

Sticks are made from sun-cured tobacco known as brus and wrapped in cigarette paper.

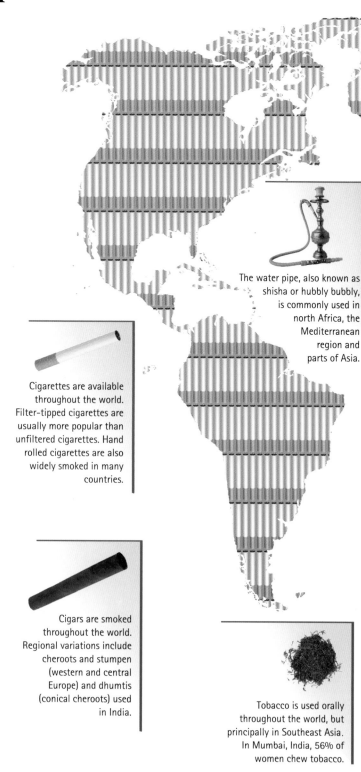

The water pipe, also known as shisha or hubbly bubbly, is commonly used in north Africa, the Mediterranean region and parts of Asia.

Cigarettes are available throughout the world. Filter-tipped cigarettes are usually more popular than unfiltered cigarettes. Hand rolled cigarettes are also widely smoked in many countries.

Cigars are smoked throughout the world. Regional variations include cheroots and stumpen (western and central Europe) and dhumtis (conical cheroots) used in India.

Tobacco is used orally throughout the world, but principally in Southeast Asia. In Mumbai, India, 56% of women chew tobacco.

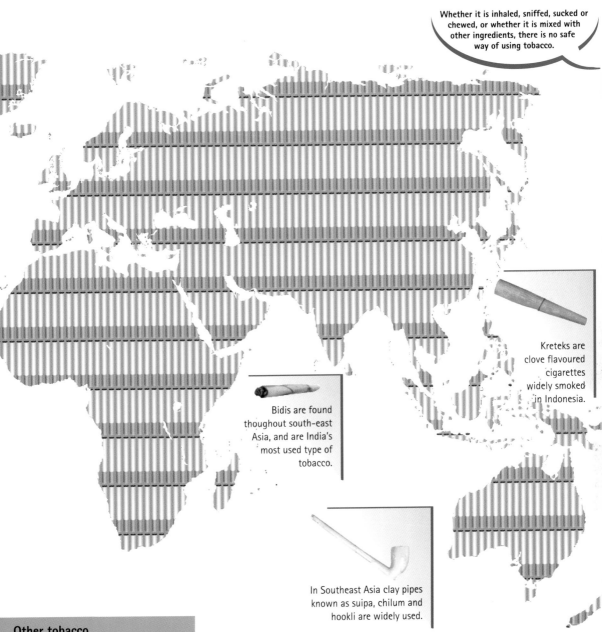

Whether it is inhaled, sniffed, sucked or chewed, or whether it is mixed with other ingredients, there is no safe way of using tobacco.

Kreteks are clove flavoured cigarettes widely smoked in Indonesia.

Bidis are found thoughout south-east Asia, and are India's most used type of tobacco.

In Southeast Asia clay pipes known as suipa, chilum and hookli are widely used.

Other tobacco

Chewing tobacco is also known as plug, loose-leaf, and twist. Pan masala, or betel quid consists of tobacco, areca nuts and staked lime wrapped in a betel leaf. They can also contain other sweetenings and flavouring agents. Varieties of pan include kaddipudi,hogesoppu, gundi, kadapam, zarda, pattiwala, kiwam, mishri, and pills.

Moist snuff is taken orally. A small amount of ground tobacco is held in the mouth between the cheek and gum. Increasingly manufacturers are pre-packaging moist snuff into small paper or cloth packets, to make the product easier to use. Other products include khaini, shammaah and nass or naswa.

Dry snuff is powdered tobacco that is inhaled through the nose or taken by mouth. Once widespread, its use is now in decline.

23

Male Smoking

Smoking has been portrayed by its sellers as a manly, masculine habit, linked to health, happiness, fitness, wealth, power and sexual success. In reality, it leads to sickness, premature death and sexual problems.

Almost one billion men in the world smoke – about 35 percent of men in developed countries and 50 percent of men in developing countries. Trends in both developed and developing countries show that male smoking rates have now peaked and, slowly but surely, are declining. However, this is an extremely slow trend over decades, and in the meantime men are dying in their millions from tobacco. In general, the educated man is giving up the habit first, so that smoking is becoming a habit of poorer, less educated males.

China deserves special mention because of the enormity of the problem. Comprising over 300 million male smokers, this huge market is, according to Philip Morris, "the most important feature on the landscape."

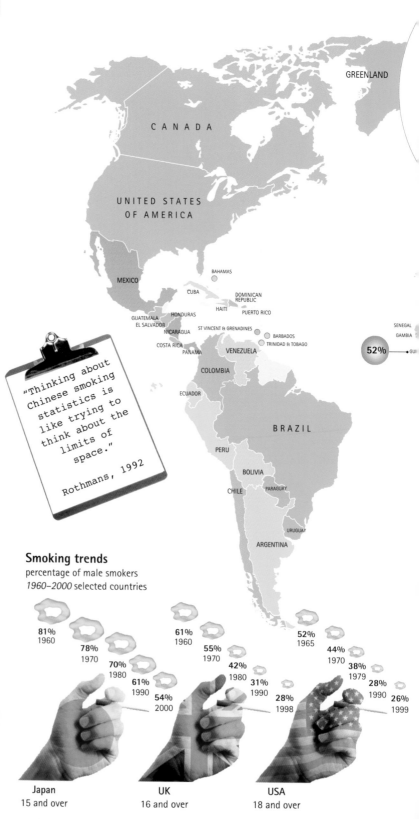

"Thinking about Chinese smoking statistics is like trying to think about the limits of space."

Rothmans, 1992

over 300 million

men in China
– equal to the
entire population
of the USA –
are smokers

Smoking trends
percentage of male smokers
1960–2000 selected countries

Japan
15 and over

- 81% 1960
- 78% 1970
- 70% 1980
- 61% 1990
- 54% 2000

UK
16 and over

- 61% 1960
- 55% 1970
- 42% 1980
- 31% 1990
- 28% 1998

USA
18 and over

- 52% 1965
- 44% 1970
- 38% 1979
- 28% 1990
- 26% 1999

52%

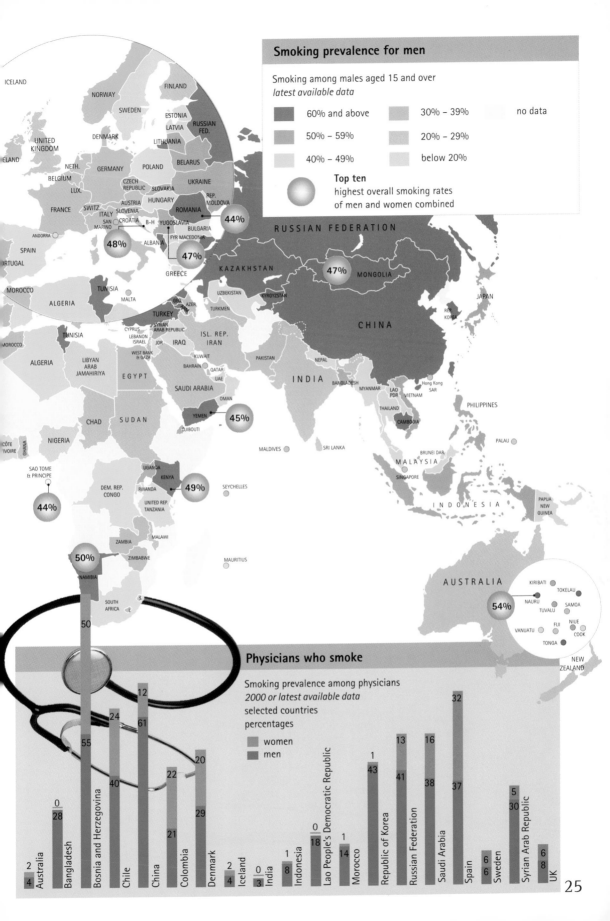

Smoking prevalence for men

Smoking among males aged 15 and over
latest available data

- 60% and above
- 50% – 59%
- 40% – 49%
- 30% – 39%
- 20% – 29%
- below 20%
- no data

Top ten
highest overall smoking rates
of men and women combined

Top ten markers: 48%, 47%, 44%, 47%, 45%, 49%, 44%, 50%, 54%

Physicians who smoke

Smoking prevalence among physicians
2000 or latest available data
selected countries
percentages

- women
- men

Country	women	men
Australia	2	4
Bangladesh	0	28
Bosnia and Herzegovina	55	40
Chile	24	61
China	12	
Colombia	22	21
Denmark	20	29
Iceland	2	4
India	0	3
Indonesia	1	8
Lao People's Democratic Republic	0	18
Morocco	1	14
Republic of Korea	1	43
Russian Federation	13	41
Saudi Arabia	16	38
Spain	32	37
Sweden	6	6
Syrian Arab Republic	5	30
UK	6	8

50

25

4 | Female Smoking

About 250 million women in the world are daily smokers. About 22 percent of women in developed countries and 9 percent of women in developing countries smoke tobacco. In addition, many women in south Asia chew tobacco.

Cigarette smoking among women is declining in many developed countries, notably Australia, Canada, the UK and the USA. But this trend is not found in all developed countries. In several southern, central and eastern European countries cigarette smoking is either still increasing among women or has not shown any decline.

The tobacco industry promotes cigarettes to women using seductive but false images of vitality, slimness, modernity, emancipation, sophistication, and sexual allure. In reality, it causes disease and death. Tobacco companies have now produced a range of brands aimed at women. Most notable are the "women-only" brands: these "feminised" cigarettes are long, extra-slim, low-tar, light-coloured or menthol.

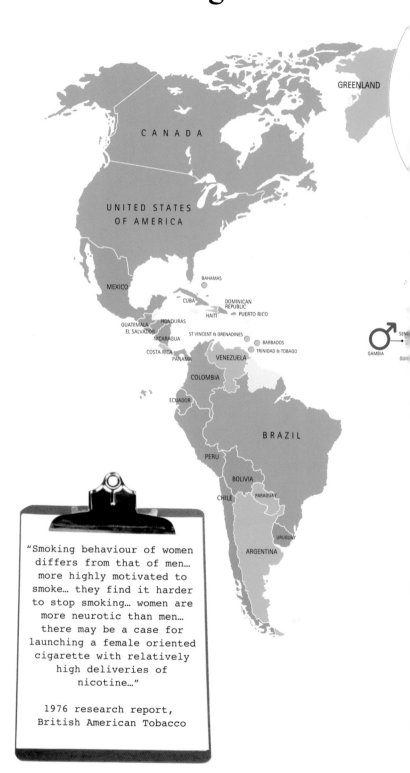

"Smoking behaviour of women differs from that of men... more highly motivated to smoke... they find it harder to stop smoking... women are more neurotic than men... there may be a case for launching a female oriented cigarette with relatively high deliveries of nicotine..."

1976 research report, British American Tobacco

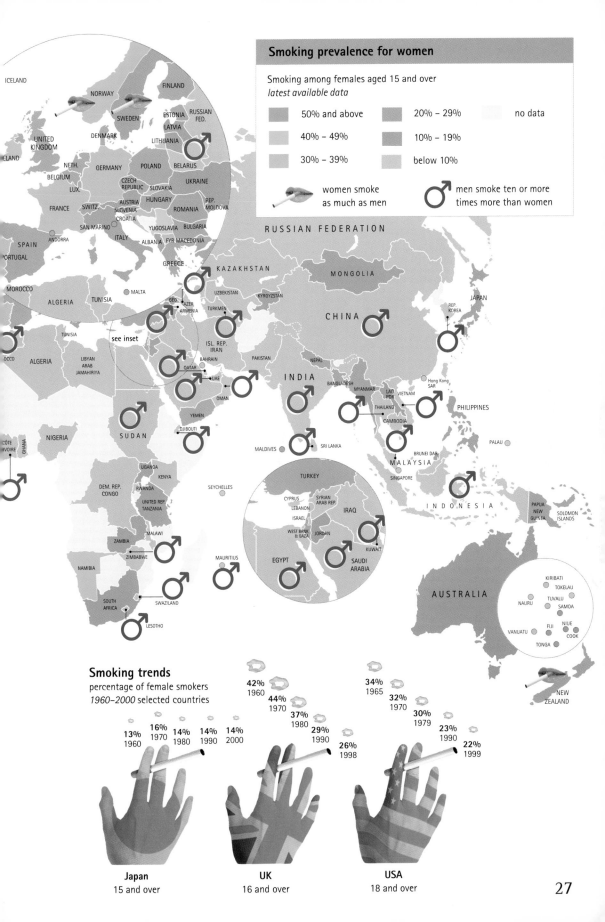

Smoking prevalence for women

Smoking among females aged 15 and over
latest available data

50% and above	20% – 29%
40% – 49%	10% – 19%
30% – 39%	below 10%
	no data

women smoke
as much as men

men smoke ten or more
times more than women

Smoking trends
percentage of female smokers
1960–2000 selected countries

Japan
15 and over

13% 1960
16% 1970
14% 1980
14% 1990
14% 2000

UK
16 and over

42% 1960
44% 1970
37% 1980
29% 1990
26% 1998

USA
18 and over

34% 1965
32% 1970
30% 1979
23% 1990
22% 1999

27

Youth

The overwhelming majority of smokers begin tobacco use before they reach adulthood. Among those young people who smoke, nearly one-quarter smoked their first cigarette before they reached the age of ten.

Several factors increase the risk of youth smoking. These include tobacco industry advertising and promotion, easy access to tobacco products, and low prices. Peer pressure plays an important role through friends' and siblings' smoking. Other risk factors associated with youth smoking include having a lower self-image than peers, and perceiving that tobacco use is normal or "cool". Many studies show that parental smoking is associated with higher youth smoking.

While the most serious effects of tobacco use normally occur after decades of smoking, there are also immediate negative health effects for young smokers. Most teenage smokers are already addicted while in adolescence. The younger a person begins to smoke, the greater the risk of eventually contracting smoking-caused diseases such as cancer or heart disease.

The highest youth smoking rates can be found in Central and Eastern Europe, sections of India, and some of the Western Pacific islands.

Fewer than 5% of young people in Bahamas, Barbados, Costa Rica, Indonesia, Malawi, Montserrat, Poland, Russia, Singapore, Ukraine and Venezuela think girls who smoke look more attractive.

Over 40% of young people in Fiji, Ghana, Malawi, Nigeria, South Africa, Sri Lanka and Zimbabwe think boys who smoke have more friends.

50%
of young people who continue to smoke will die from smoking

Early smokers
Over 30% of children smoked their first whole cigarette before age 10 in Ghana, Grenada, Guyana, India, Jamaica, Palau, Poland, N Mariana Islands and St Lucia.

"It is important to know as much as possible about teenage smoking patterns and attitudes. Today's teenager is tomorrow's potential regular customer, and the overwhelming majority of smokers first begin to smoke while still in their teens... The smoking patterns of teenagers are particularly important to Philip Morris."

Philip Morris Companies Inc.
1981

40%
of children worldwide are exposed to passive smoking at home

BOYS

C A N A D A

UNITED STATES
OF AMERICA

MEXICO

BAHAMAS
CUBA
JAMAICA
HAITI
MONSERRAT
GRENADA
VENEZUELA
COSTA RICA

ANTIGUA & BARBUDA
DOMINICA
BARBADOS
TRINIDAD & TOBAGO
GUYANA
SURINAME

PERU
BOLIVIA
CHILE

URUGUAY
ARGENTINA

POLAND
UKRAINE

RUSSIAN FEDERATION

CHINA

JORDAN

NEPAL

INDIA

GHANA
NIGERIA

KENYA

MALAWI
ZIMBABWE

SOUTH
AFRICA

SRI LANKA

SINGAPORE

NORTHERN
MARIANA
ISLANDS

PHILIPPINES

PALAU

INDONESIA

FIJI

Tobacco users

Percentage of 13–15 year olds
using tobacco
*2001 or latest available
national, regional or city data*

- 30% and over
- 20% – 29%
- 10% – 19%
- under 10%
- variable 3% – 60%
- no data

RUSSIAN FEDERATION

POLAND
UKRAINE

UNITED STATES
OF AMERICA

MEXICO
CUBA
JAMAICA
HAITI
MONSERRAT
GRENADA
VENEZUELA
COSTA RICA

BAHAMAS

ANTIGUA & BARBUDA
DOMINICA
BARBADOS
TRINIDAD & TOBAGO
GUYANA
SURINAME

PERU
BOLIVIA
CHILE

URUGUAY
ARGENTINA

JORDAN

CHINA

NEPAL

INDIA

GHANA
NIGERIA

KENYA

MALAWI
ZIMBABWE

SOUTH
AFRICA

SRI LANKA

SINGAPORE

NORTHERN
MARIANA
ISLANDS

PHILIPPINES

PALAU

INDONESIA

FIJI

GIRLS

Cigarette Consumption

Global consumption of cigarettes has been rising steadily since manufactured cigarettes were introduced at the beginning of the 20th century. While consumption is levelling off and even decreasing in some countries, worldwide more people are smoking, and smokers are smoking more cigarettes.

The numbers of smokers will increase mainly due to expansion of the world's population. By 2030 there will be at least another 2 billion people in the world. Even if prevalence rates fall, the absolute number of smokers will increase. The expected continuing decrease in male smoking prevalence will be offset by the increase in female smoking rates, especially in developing countries.

The consumption of tobacco has reached the proportions of a global epidemic. Tobacco companies are cranking out cigarettes at the rate of five and a half trillion a year – nearly 1,000 cigarettes for every man, woman, and child on the planet.

Cigarettes account for the largest share of manufactured tobacco products, 96 percent of total value sales. Asia, Australia and the Far East are by far the largest consumers (2,715 billion cigarettes), followed by the Americas (745 billion), Eastern Europe and Former Soviet Economies (631 billion) and Western Europe (606 billion).

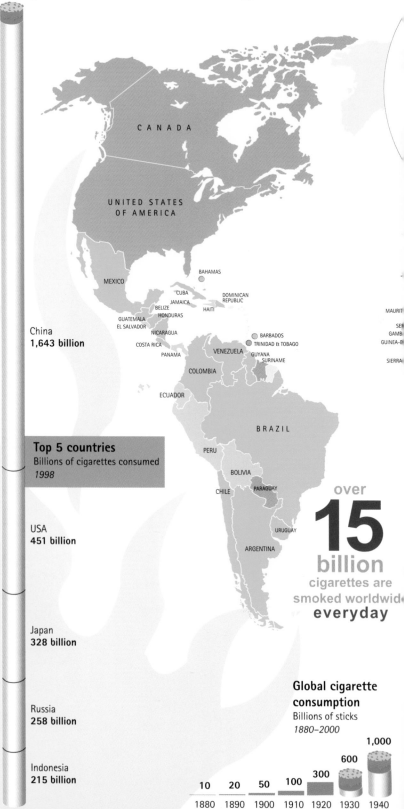

China
1,643 billion

Top 5 countries
Billions of cigarettes consumed
1998

USA
451 billion

Japan
328 billion

Russia
258 billion

Indonesia
215 billion

over

15
billion
cigarettes are
smoked worldwide
everyday

**Global cigarette
consumption**
Billions of sticks
1880–2000

						1,000
				300	600	
10	20	50	100			
1880	1890	1900	1910	1920	1930	1940

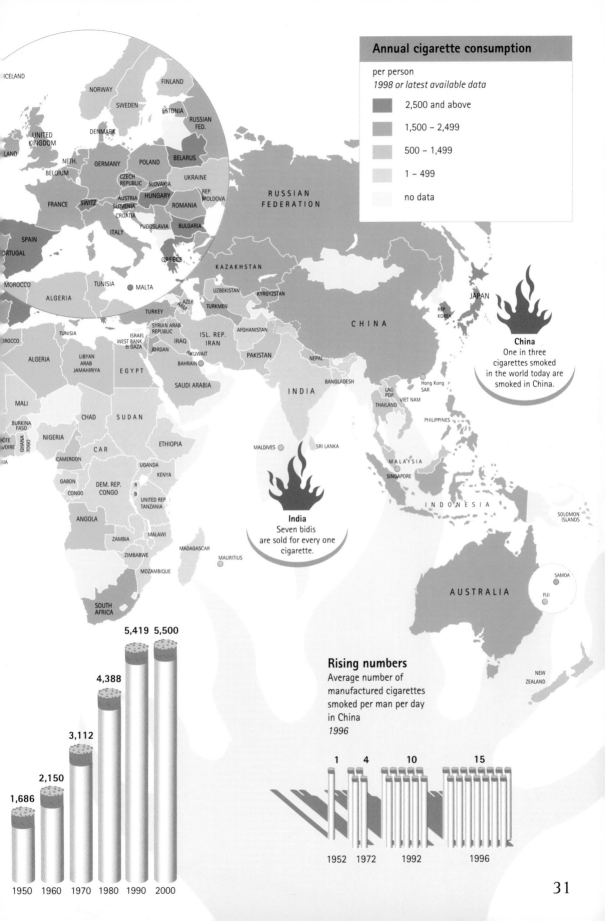

Annual cigarette consumption

per person
1998 or latest available data

- 2,500 and above
- 1,500 – 2,499
- 500 – 1,499
- 1 – 499
- no data

China
One in three cigarettes smoked in the world today are smoked in China.

India
Seven bidis are sold for every one cigarette.

5,419 5,500

4,388

3,112

2,150

1,686

1950 1960 1970 1980 1990 2000

Rising numbers
Average number of manufactured cigarettes smoked per man per day in China
1996

1   4   10   15

1952 1972   1992   1996

31

Health Risks

Tobacco is packed with harmful and addictive substances. Scientific evidence has shown conclusively that all forms of tobacco cause health problems throughout life, frequently resulting in death or disability.

Smokers have markedly increased risks of multiple cancers, particularly lung cancer, and are at far greater risk of heart disease, strokes, emphysema and many other fatal and non-fatal diseases. If they chew tobacco, they risk cancer of the lip, tongue and mouth.

Women suffer additional health risks. Smoking in pregnancy is dangerous to the mother as well as to the foetus, especially in poor countries where health facilities are inadequate.

Maternal smoking is not only harmful during pregnancy, but has long-term effects on the baby after birth. This is often compounded by exposure to passive smoking from the mother, father or other adults smoking.

While tobacco kills millions more than it helps, research is underway examining any possible health benefits of nicotine and also trying to find a safe use for tobacco, particularly in the field of genetic modification. The aim is to produce vaccines or human proteins for medical use, or even to clean up soil that has been contaminated with explosives.

Deadly chemicals

Tobacco smoke contains over 4,000 chemicals, some of which have marked irritant properties and some 60 are known or suspected carcinogens.

Tobacco smoke includes	as found in
Acetone	paint stripper
Ammonia	floor cleaner
Arsenic	ant poison
Butane	lighter fuel
Cadmium	car batteries
Carbon monoxide	car exhaust fumes
DDT	insecticide
Hydrogen cyanide	gas chambers
Methanol	rocket fuel
Napthalene	moth balls
Toluene	industrial solvent
Vinyl chloride	plastics

Babes in the womb
Smoking in pregnancy

Increased risks:
Spontaneous abortion / miscarriage
Ectopic pregnancy
Abruptio placentae
Placenta praevia
Premature rupture of the membranes
Premature birth

Foetus:
Smaller infant (for gestational age)
Stillborn infant
Birth defects, eg congenital limb reduction
Increased nicotine receptors in baby's brain
Increased likelihood of
infant smoking as a teenager
Possible physical and mental
long-term effects

Time ticks away

Every cigarette takes 7 minutes off your life

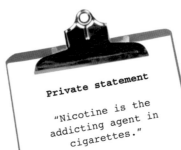

Private statement

"Nicotine is the addicting agent in cigarettes."

Brown & Williamson official in 1983

Sworn testimony

"I believe that nicotine is not addictive."

CEOs of the seven leading tobacco companies in 1994

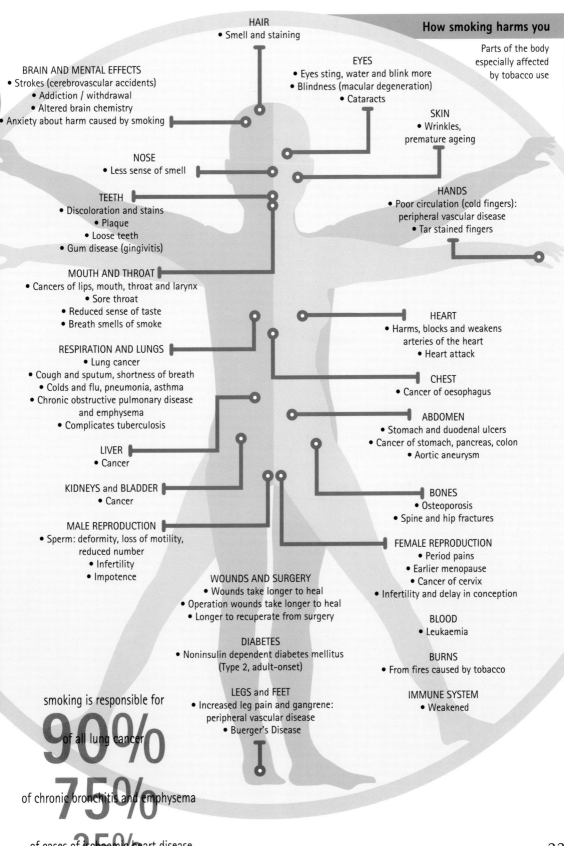

HAIR
• Smell and staining

How smoking harms you

Parts of the body
especially affected
by tobacco use

EYES
• Eyes sting, water and blink more
• Blindness (macular degeneration)
• Cataracts

BRAIN AND MENTAL EFFECTS
• Strokes (cerebrovascular accidents)
• Addiction / withdrawal
• Altered brain chemistry
• Anxiety about harm caused by smoking

SKIN
• Wrinkles,
premature ageing

NOSE
• Less sense of smell

TEETH
• Discoloration and stains
• Plaque
• Loose teeth
• Gum disease (gingivitis)

HANDS
• Poor circulation (cold fingers):
peripheral vascular disease
• Tar stained fingers

MOUTH AND THROAT
• Cancers of lips, mouth, throat and larynx
• Sore throat
• Reduced sense of taste
• Breath smells of smoke

HEART
• Harms, blocks and weakens
arteries of the heart
• Heart attack

RESPIRATION AND LUNGS
• Lung cancer
• Cough and sputum, shortness of breath
• Colds and flu, pneumonia, asthma
• Chronic obstructive pulmonary disease
and emphysema
• Complicates tuberculosis

CHEST
• Cancer of oesophagus

ABDOMEN
• Stomach and duodenal ulcers
• Cancer of stomach, pancreas, colon
• Aortic aneurysm

LIVER
• Cancer

KIDNEYS and BLADDER
• Cancer

BONES
• Osteoporosis
• Spine and hip fractures

MALE REPRODUCTION
• Sperm: deformity, loss of motility,
reduced number
• Infertility
• Impotence

FEMALE REPRODUCTION
• Period pains
• Earlier menopause
• Cancer of cervix
• Infertility and delay in conception

WOUNDS AND SURGERY
• Wounds take longer to heal
• Operation wounds take longer to heal
• Longer to recuperate from surgery

BLOOD
• Leukaemia

DIABETES
• Noninsulin dependent diabetes mellitus
(Type 2, adult–onset)

BURNS
• From fires caused by tobacco

LEGS and FEET
• Increased leg pain and gangrene:
peripheral vascular disease
• Buerger's Disease

IMMUNE SYSTEM
• Weakened

smoking is responsible for

90%
of all lung cancer

75%
of chronic bronchitis and emphysema

25%
of cases of ischaemic heart disease

33

Passive Smoking

The first conclusive evidence on the danger of passive smoking came from Takeshi Hirayama's study in 1981 on lung cancer in non-smoking Japanese women married to men who smoked. Although the tobacco industry immediately launched a multi-million dollar campaign to discredit the evidence, dozens of further studies have confirmed the link. Research then broadened into other areas and new scientific evidence continues to accumulate.

A complex mixture of chemicals is generated from the burning and smoking of tobacco. As a passive smoker, the non-smoker breathes "sidestream" smoke from the burning tip of the cigarette and "mainstream" smoke that has been inhaled and then exhaled by the smoker.

The risk of lung cancer in non-smokers exposed to passive smoking is increased by between 20 and 30 percent, and the excess risk of heart disease is 23 percent.

Children are at particular risk from adults' smoking. Adverse health effects include pneumonia and bronchitis, coughing and wheezing, worsening of asthma, middle ear disease, and possibly neuro-behavioural impairment and cardiovascular disease in adulthood.

A pregnant woman's exposure to other people's smoking can harm her foetus. The effects are compounded when the child is exposed to passive smoking after birth.

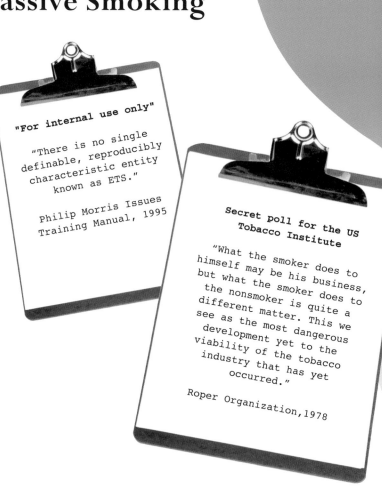

"For internal use only"

"There is no single definable, reproducibly characteristic entity known as ETS."

Philip Morris Issues Training Manual, 1995

Secret poll for the US Tobacco Institute

"What the smoker does to himself may be his business, but what the smoker does to the nonsmoker is quite a different matter. This we see as the most dangerous development yet to the viability of the tobacco industry that has yet occurred."

Roper Organization, 1978

Children exposed to passive smoking at home

selected countries
2001 or latest available data
percentages

Country	%
Cuba	69%
Argentina	68%
Poland	67%
Indonesia	63%
Chile	57%
Russian Federation	55%
China	53%
Ukraine	49%
Bolivia	46%
Mexico	45.5%
India	34%
Nigeria	34%
Haiti	31%
Peru	29%

Harm caused by passive smoking

Health effects on adults

HAIR
- Smell

BRAIN AND MENTAL EFFECTS
- Strokes

EYES
- Sting, water and blink more

NOSE
- Irritation

RESPIRATION AND LUNGS
- Lung cancer
- Worsening of pre-existing chest problems, such as asthma, chronic obstructive pulmonary disease and emphysema

HEART
- Harms, clogs weakens arteries
- Heart attack, angina

UTERUS
- Low birthweight or small for gestational age
- Cot death or Sudden Infant Death Syndrome (SIDS) after birth

BURNS
- From fires caused by tobacco

Harm caused by passive smoking

Health effects on children

HAIR
- Smell

BRAIN
- Possible association with brain tumours and long-term mental effects

EYES
- Sting, water and blink more

EARS
- Middle ear infections (chronic otitis media)

RESPIRATION AND LUNGS
- Respiratory infections (including bronchitis and pneumonia)
- Asthma induction and exacerbation
- Chronic respiratory symptoms (wheezing, cough, breathlessness)
- Decreased lung function

HEART
- Deleterious effects on oxygen, arteries
- Increased nicotine receptors

BLOOD
- Possible association with lymphoma

BURNS
- From fires caused by tobacco

ROLE MODEL
- Greater likelihood of becoming a smoker as a teenager

Numbers affected by passive smoking in the USA
annual *1990s*

Lung cancer 3,000
Ischaemic heart disease 35,000 to 62,000

Infants and children

Low birthweight 9,700 to 18,600
Cot death (SIDS) 1,900 to 2,700
Bronchitis or pneumonia in infants 150,000 to 300,000

Respiratory effects in children
Middle ear infection 700,000 to 1,600,000
Asthma induction (new cases) 8,000 to 26,000
Asthma exacerbation 400,000 to 1,000,000

9 Deaths

Cigarettes kill half of all lifetime users. Half die in middle age – between 35 and 69 years old.

No other consumer product is as dangerous, or kills as many people. Tobacco kills more than AIDS, legal drugs, illegal drugs, road accidents, murder, and suicide combined.

Tobacco already kills more men in developing countries than in industrialised countries, and it is likely that deaths among women will soon be the same.

While 0.1 billion people died from tobacco use in the 20th century, ten times as many will die in the 21st century. Maternal smoking during pregnancy is responsible for many foetal deaths and is also a major cause of Sudden Infant Death Syndrome.

Passive smoking in the home, workplace, or in public places also kills, although in lower numbers. However, those killed do not die from their own habit, but from someone else's. Children are at particular risk from adults smoking, and even smoking by other adults around a pregnant woman has a harmful effect on a foetus.

"...with a general lengthening of the expectation of life we really need something for people to die of..."

Report for Tobacco Advisory Council, 1978

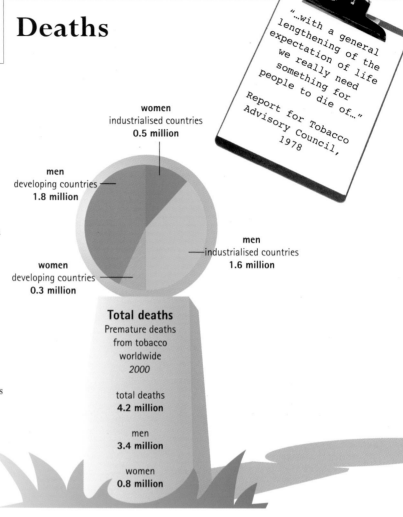

women
industrialised countries
0.5 million

men
developing countries
1.8 million

men
industrialised countries
1.6 million

women
developing countries
0.3 million

Total deaths
Premature deaths
from tobacco
worldwide
2000

total deaths
4.2 million

men
3.4 million

women
0.8 million

of everyone alive today

500,000,000

will eventually be killed by tobacco

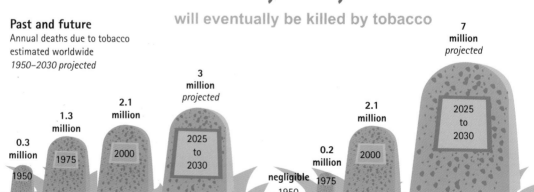

Past and future
Annual deaths due to tobacco
estimated worldwide
1950–2030 projected

0.3 million
1950

1.3 million
1975

2.1 million
2000

3 million
projected
2025 to 2030

negligible
1950

0.2 million
1975

2.1 million
2000

7 million
projected
2025 to 2030

industrialised countries

developing countries

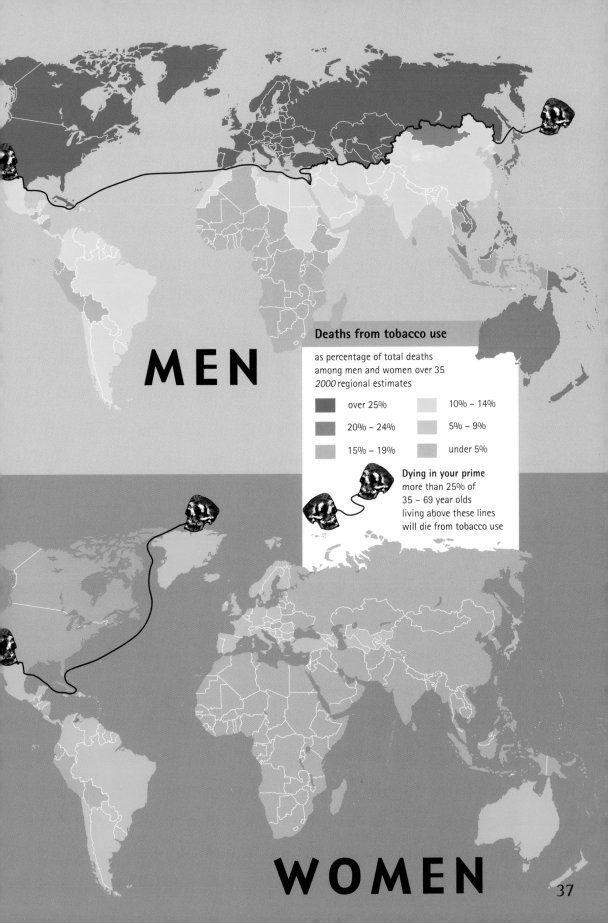

MEN

WOMEN

Deaths from tobacco use

as percentage of total deaths
among men and women over 35
2000 regional estimates

- over 25%
- 20% – 24%
- 15% – 19%
- 10% – 14%
- 5% – 9%
- under 5%

Dying in your prime
more than 25% of
35 – 69 year olds
living above these lines
will die from tobacco use

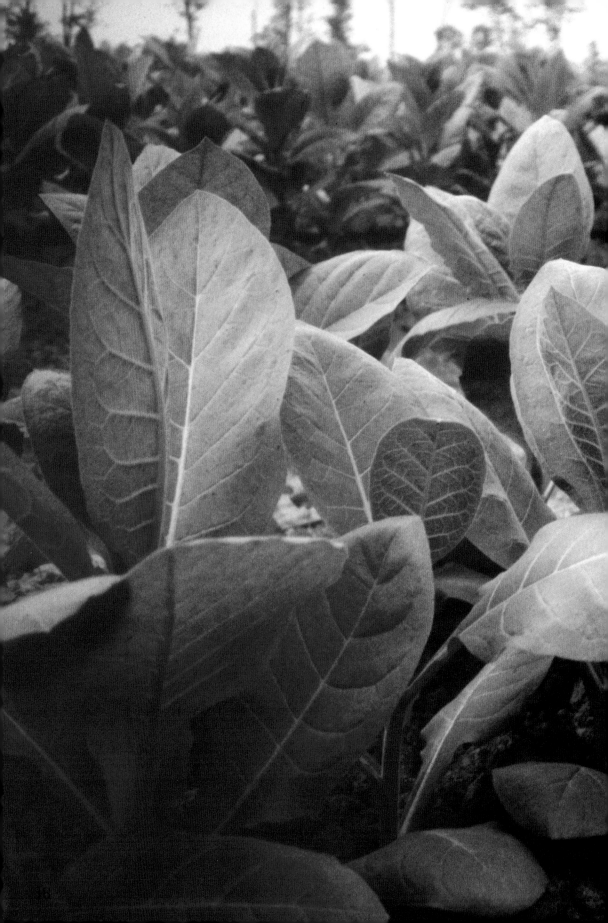

PART 2

THE COSTS OF TOBACCO

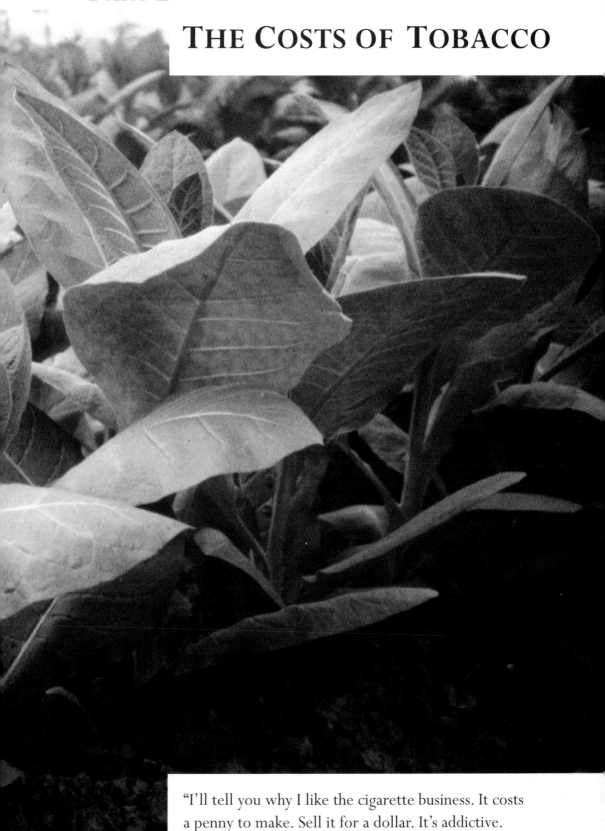

"I'll tell you why I like the cigarette business. It costs
a penny to make. Sell it for a dollar. It's addictive.
And there's fantastic brand loyalty."

Warren Buffet, investor, 1990s

Costs to the Economy

The tobacco industry uses economic arguments to persuade governments, the media and the general population that smoking benefits the economy. It claims that if tobacco control measures are introduced, tax revenues will fall, jobs will be lost and there will be great hardship to the economy.

But the industry greatly exaggerates the economic losses, if any, which tobacco control measures will cause and they never mention the economic costs which tobacco inflicts upon every country.

Tobacco's cost to governments, to employers and to the environment includes social, welfare and health care spending, loss of foreign exchange in importing cigarettes; loss of land that could grow food; costs of fires and damage to buildings caused by careless smoking; environmental costs ranging from deforestation to collection of smokers' litter, absenteeism, decreased productivity, higher numbers of accidents and higher insurance premiums.

Smoking accounted for over

6%

of total health care expenses in the USA in 1999

Canada $1.6 billion

USA $76 billion

Health-care cost

Health care cost attributable to tobacco 2002 or latest available estimate selected countries

Average days off sick per year in the USA 2001

6.16 smokers
4.53 ex-smokers
3.86 never-smokers

"...reflecting 5.23 years of life lost for the average smoker — indirect positive effects [are that] public finance benefits from smoking indirectly, via savings on the health care costs — in pensions — and public housing costs savings."

Report on the Czech Republic, commissioned by Philip Morris, 2001

"Philip Morris Apologizes for Report Touting Benefits of Smokers's Deaths."

Wall Street Journal headline, 2001

Trash collected in the USA
43 states 1996

cigarette butts **20%**

other **80%**

40

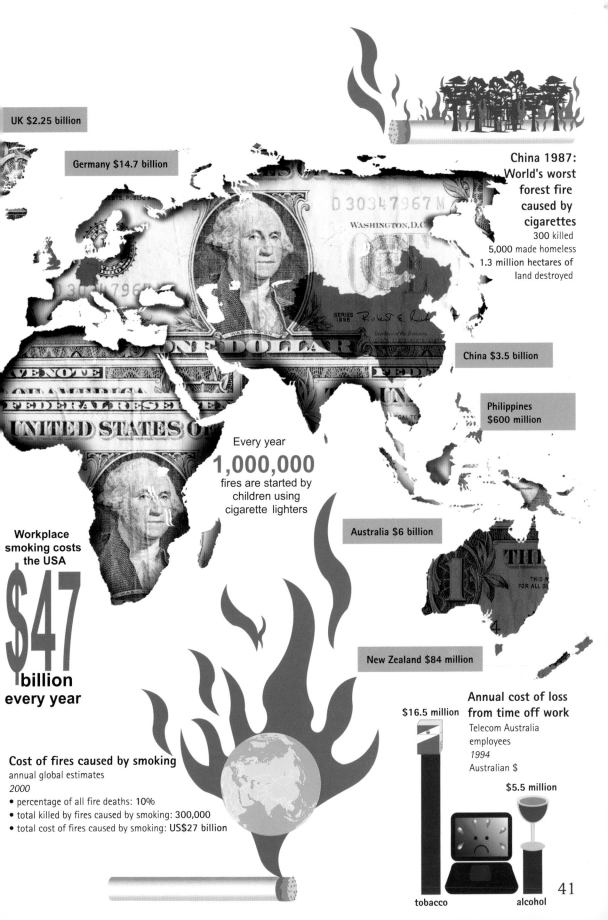

UK $2.25 billion

Germany $14.7 billion

China 1987: World's worst forest fire caused by cigarettes
300 killed
5,000 made homeless
1.3 million hectares of land destroyed

China $3.5 billion

Philippines $600 million

Every year
1,000,000
fires are started by children using cigarette lighters

Australia $6 billion

Workplace smoking costs the USA

$47 billion every year

New Zealand $84 million

Cost of fires caused by smoking
annual global estimates
2000
• percentage of all fire deaths: 10%
• total killed by fires caused by smoking: 300,000
• total cost of fires caused by smoking: US$27 billion

$16.5 million

Annual cost of loss from time off work
Telecom Australia employees
1994
Australian $

$5.5 million

tobacco   alcohol

41

11 | Costs to the Smoker

The economic costs of smoking to smokers and their families include money spent on buying tobacco, which could otherwise be used on food, clothing and shelter, family holidays or a car.

As smoking kills a quarter of all smokers in their working years, smoking deprives the smoker's family of many years of income. Smokers also suffer loss of income through illness. Following a smoker's premature death, a partner, children or elderly parents can be left destitute.

Family members of smokers lose income through time taken looking after smokers when they are sick, and time lost taking them to hospital. In some developing countries a hospital visit can take days.

Smokers also have to shoulder higher health insurance premiums, and many other miscellaneous costs, such as increased wear and tear on their home, as well as increased fire risk.

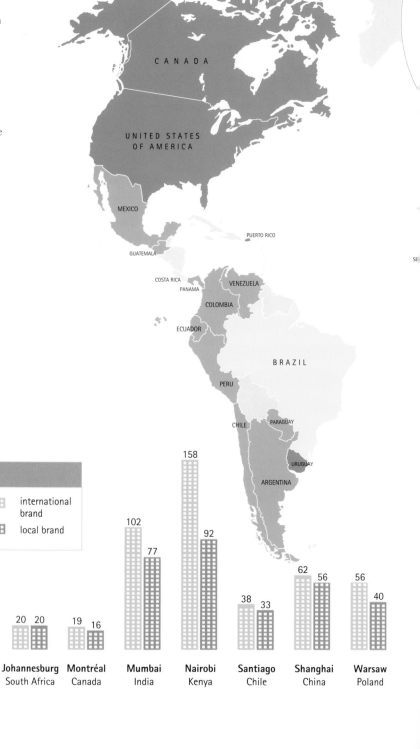

A hard day's smoke

Minutes of labour worked to purchase 20 cigarettes
2000 selected cities

- international brand
- local brand

Abu Dhabi United Arab Emirates	**Copenhagen** Denmark	**Jakarta** Indonesia	**Johannesburg** South Africa	**Montréal** Canada	**Mumbai** India	**Nairobi** Kenya	**Santiago** Chile	**Shanghai** China	**Warsaw** Poland
20 / 11	23 / 23	62 / 62	20 / 20	19 / 16	102 / 77	158 / 92	38 / 33	62 / 56	56 / 40

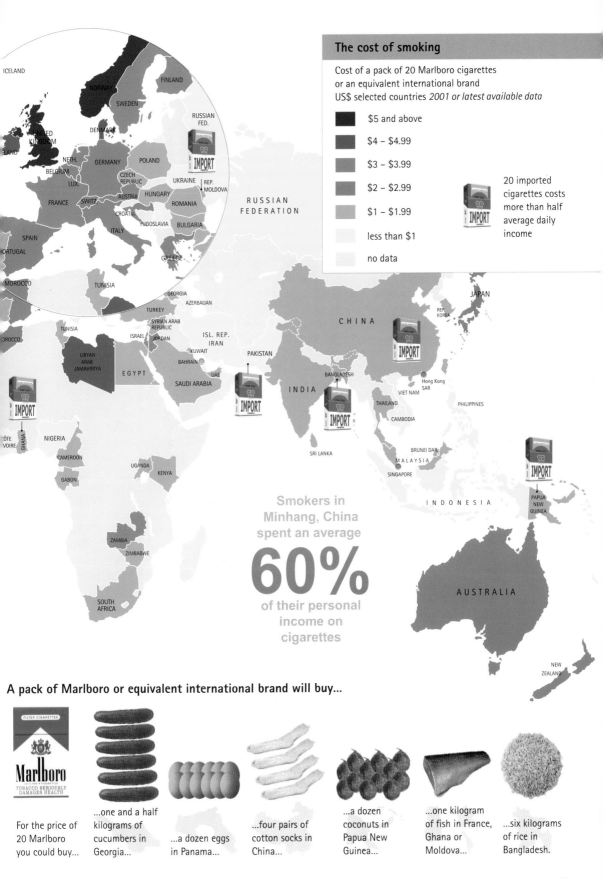

The cost of smoking

Cost of a pack of 20 Marlboro cigarettes
or an equivalent international brand
US$ selected countries *2001 or latest available data*

- $5 and above
- $4 – $4.99
- $3 – $3.99
- $2 – $2.99
- $1 – $1.99
- less than $1
- no data

20 imported cigarettes costs more than half average daily income

RUSSIAN FEDERATION

MOROCCO
TUNISIA
GEORGIA
AZERBAIJAN
TURKEY
SYRIAN ARAB REPUBLIC
ISRAEL
JORDAN
ISL. REP. IRAN
KUWAIT
BAHRAIN
UAE
LIBYAN ARAB JAMAHIRIYA
EGYPT
SAUDI ARABIA
PAKISTAN
BANGLADESH
INDIA
CHINA
JAPAN
REP. KOREA
Hong Kong SAR
VIET NAM
THAILAND
PHILIPPINES
CAMBODIA
SRI LANKA
BRUNEI DAR.
MALAYSIA
SINGAPORE
INDONESIA
PAPUA NEW GUINEA

CÔTE D'IVOIRE
GHANA
NIGERIA
CAMEROON
GABON
UGANDA
KENYA
ZAMBIA
ZIMBABWE
SOUTH AFRICA

AUSTRALIA
NEW ZEALAND

Smokers in Minhang, China spent an average

60%

of their personal income on cigarettes

A pack of Marlboro or equivalent international brand will buy...

For the price of 20 Marlboro you could buy...

...one and a half kilograms of cucumbers in Georgia...

...a dozen eggs in Panama...

...four pairs of cotton socks in China...

...a dozen coconuts in Papua New Guinea...

...one kilogram of fish in France, Ghana or Moldova...

...six kilograms of rice in Bangladesh.

43

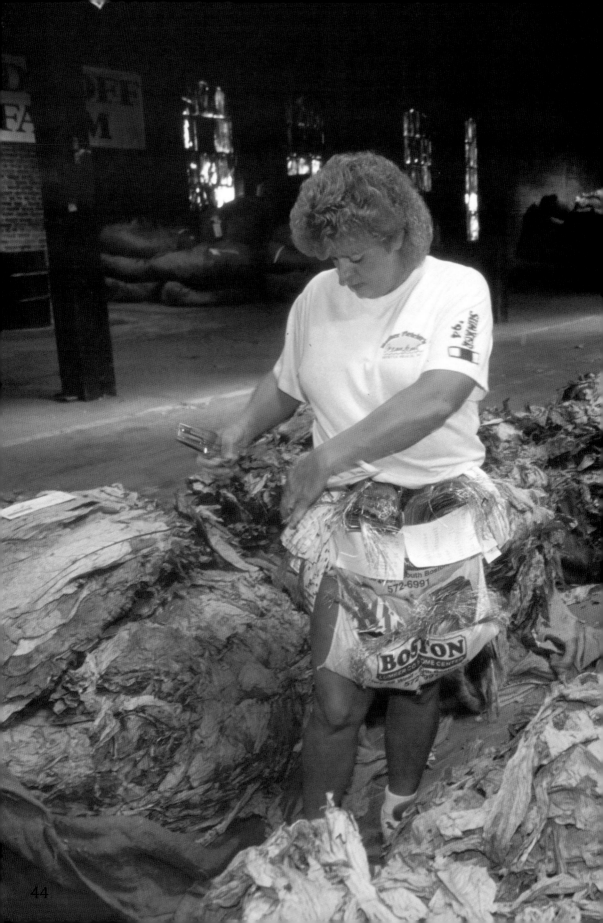

PART 3

THE TOBACCO TRADE

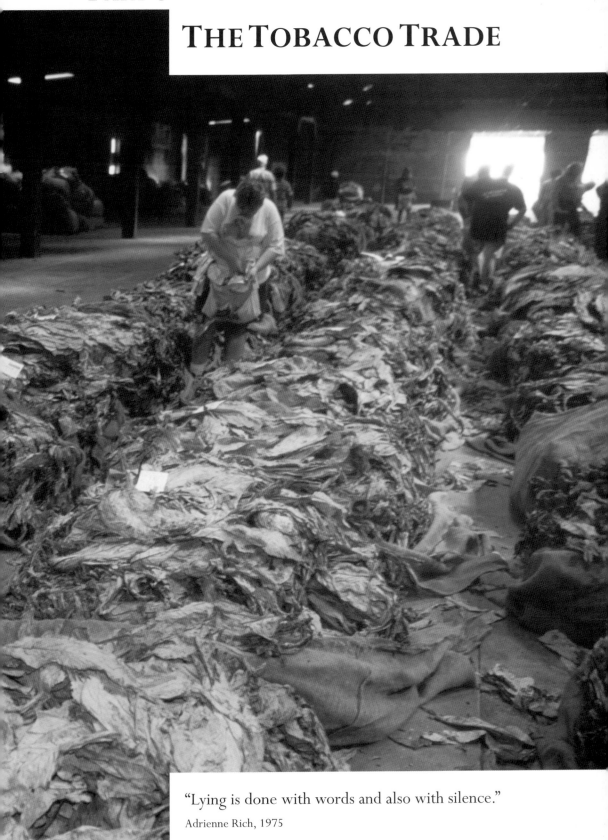

"Lying is done with words and also with silence."
Adrienne Rich, 1975

Growing Tobacco

Tobacco is grown in over 125 countries, on over 4 million hectares of land, a third of which is in China alone. The global tobacco crop is worth approximately US$20 billion, a small fraction of the total amount generated from the sale of manufactured tobacco products.

Tobacco is grown on less than one percent of the world's agricultural land, and on a wide variety of soils and climates. Since the 1960s, the bulk of production has moved from the Americas to Africa and Asia: land devoted to tobacco growing has been halved in the USA, Canada and Mexico, but has almost doubled in China, Malawi and United Republic of Tanzania.

The production of tobacco leaves has more than doubled since the 1960s, totalling nearly 7 million metric tons in 2000.

The greater use of fertilisers and pesticides, as well as the increased mechanisation, that have produced these higher yields are environmentally damaging. The problem does not end with growing tobacco: the processes used in curing tobacco leaves cause massive deforestation.

There are millions of tobacco farmers worldwide. The tobacco industry exploits them by contributing to their debt burden, while using their economic plight to argue against efforts to control tobacco. In the USA, the bond between the tobacco industry and the tobacco farmer finally is beginning to break down, and partnerships are developing between the farmers and the public health community.

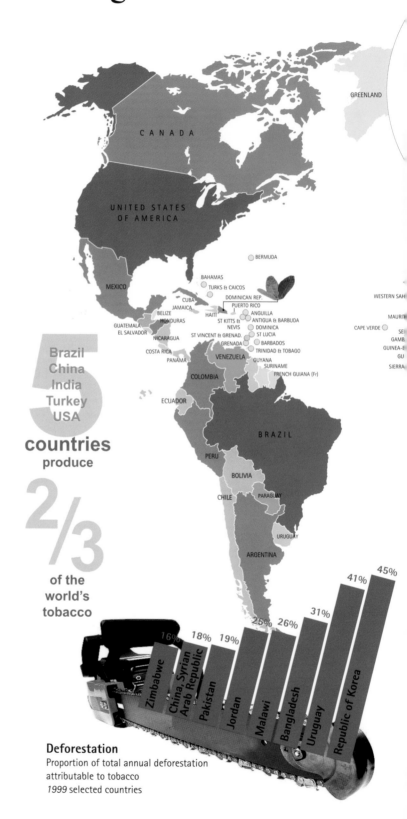

5 countries
Brazil
China
India
Turkey
USA

2/3 of the world's tobacco

Deforestation
Proportion of total annual deforestation attributable to tobacco
1999 selected countries

Zimbabwe 16%
China, Syrian Arab Republic 18%
Pakistan 19%
Jordan 25%
Malawi 26%
Bangladesh 31%
Uruguay 41%
Republic of Korea 45%

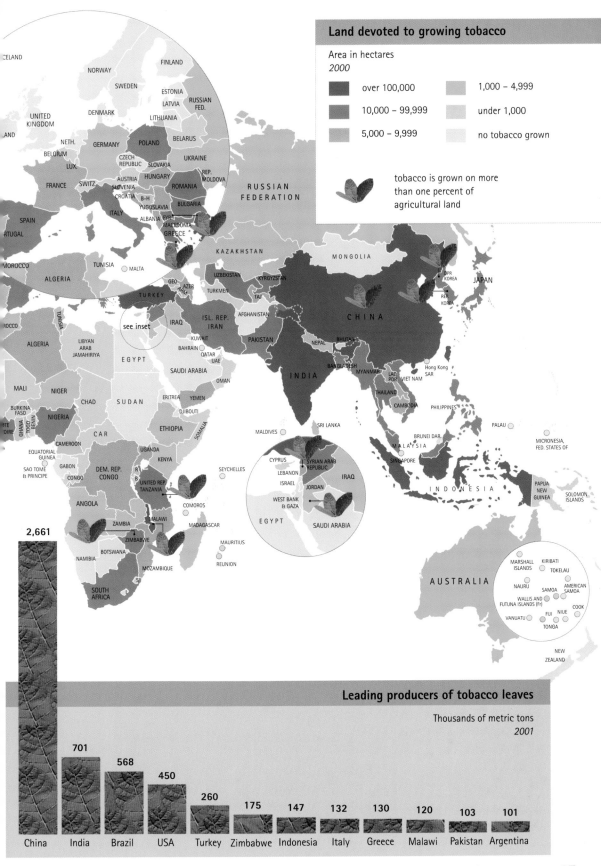

Land devoted to growing tobacco

Area in hectares
2000

- over 100,000
- 10,000 – 99,999
- 5,000 – 9,999
- 1,000 – 4,999
- under 1,000
- no tobacco grown

tobacco is grown on more than one percent of agricultural land

Leading producers of tobacco leaves

Thousands of metric tons
2001

China	India	Brazil	USA	Turkey	Zimbabwe	Indonesia	Italy	Greece	Malawi	Pakistan	Argentina
2,661	701	568	450	260	175	147	132	130	120	103	101

Each year, over five trillion cigarettes are manufactured. China is by far the largest cigarette manufacturer, followed by the USA. Chinese cigarette production increased from 225 billion cigarettes annually in 1960 to 1.7 trillion a year in 1995, a seven-fold increase. The economic value of tobacco products is vast, totalling hundreds of billions of US dollars a year. Very little of this money is spent on tobacco itself. More is spent on paper, filters, and packaging than on tobacco.

Nearly 2 million people are employed in the manufacture of tobacco products, two-thirds of whom are working in China, India and Indonesia. Job losses which would result from a reduction in tobacco consumption are estimated to be fairly small. Technological advances in both farming and manufacturing have a much larger impact on jobs than tobacco control efforts.

Hundreds of chemicals are added to tobacco in the manufacture of cigarettes. Additives make smoke easier to inhale into the lungs and allow for less tobacco to be used in each cigarette. Today's cigarettes are highly engineered, exquisitely designed "nicotine delivery devices".

Besides using less tobacco per cigarette, the composition of the cigarette is also changing. Manufacturers are using more reconstituted tobacco, which makes it easier to add chemicals and to include leaf stems and dust which had previously been discarded.

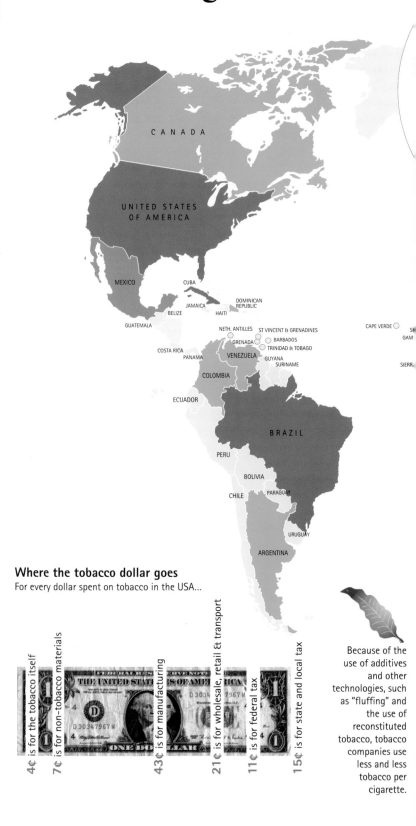

Where the tobacco dollar goes
For every dollar spent on tobacco in the USA...

4¢ is for the tobacco itself

7¢ is for non-tobacco materials

43¢ is for manufacturing

21¢ is for wholesale, retail & transport

11¢ is for federal tax

15¢ is for state and local tax

Because of the use of additives and other technologies, such as "fluffing" and the use of reconstituted tobacco, tobacco companies use less and less tobacco per cigarette.

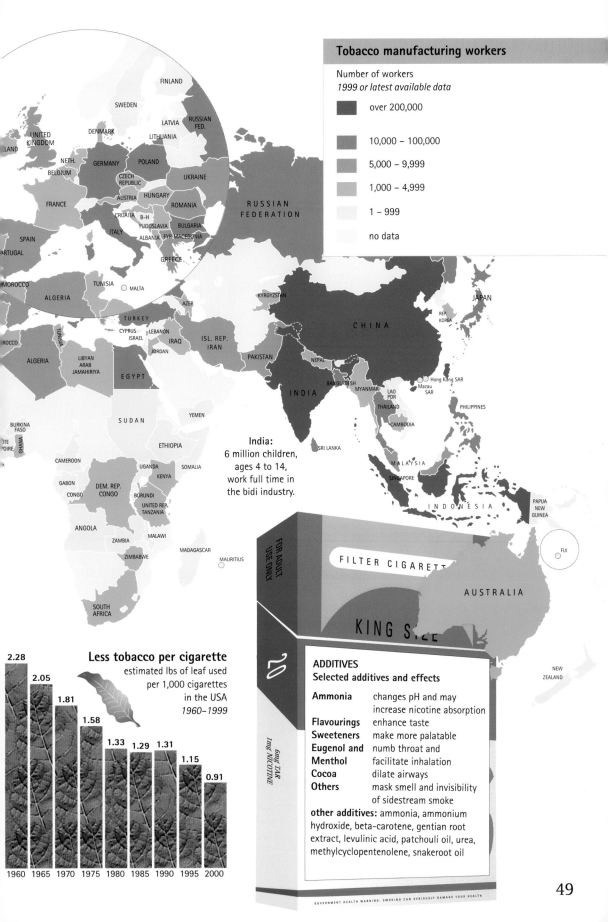

Tobacco manufacturing workers

Number of workers
1999 or latest available data

- over 200,000
- 10,000 – 100,000
- 5,000 – 9,999
- 1,000 – 4,999
- 1 – 999
- no data

India:
6 million children,
ages 4 to 14,
work full time in
the bidi industry.

Less tobacco per cigarette
estimated lbs of leaf used
per 1,000 cigarettes
in the USA
1960–1999

1960	1965	1970	1975	1980	1985	1990	1995	2000
2.28	2.05	1.81	1.58	1.33	1.29	1.31	1.15	0.91

FOR ADULT USE ONLY

FILTER CIGARETT

KING SIZE

20

6mg TAR
1mg NICOTINE

ADDITIVES
Selected additives and effects

Ammonia	changes pH and may increase nicotine absorption
Flavourings	enhance taste
Sweeteners	make more palatable
Eugenol and Menthol	numb throat and facilitate inhalation
Cocoa	dilate airways
Others	mask smell and invisibility of sidestream smoke

other additives: ammonia, ammonium
hydroxide, beta-carotene, gentian root
extract, levulinic acid, patchouli oil, urea,
methylcyclopentenolene, snakeroot oil

GOVERNMENT HEALTH WARNING: SMOKING CAN SERIOUSLY DAMAGE YOUR HEALTH

49

Tobacco Companies

Philip Morris is the world's largest transnational tobacco company, whose Marlboro brand is the world leader. In 1999 the company had sales of over US$47 billion. However, excluding the US domestic market, BAT sells the most cigarettes worldwide and has the largest network in the most countries.

The tobacco industry is a mixture of some of the most powerful transnational commercial companies in the world. Tobacco companies, which frequently merge, own other huge industries and run an intricate variety of joint ventures.

State tobacco monopolies have been in decline since the 1980s. About 7,000 medium to large state-owned enterprises were privatised in the 1980s and a further 60,000 in the 1990s after the collapse of the former Soviet Union. From the late 1990s, the IMF has pressurised countries such as the Republic of Korea, the Republic of Moldova, Thailand and Turkey to privatise their state tobacco industry as a condition of loans.

The remaining monopolies represent a combined consumption of 2 billion cigarettes or 40 percent of the world's total cigarette consumption.

Since the early 1990s, the cigarette companies have massively increased their manufacturing capacity in developing countries and eastern Europe. Where once the rich countries exported "death and disease", increasingly these are manufactured locally.

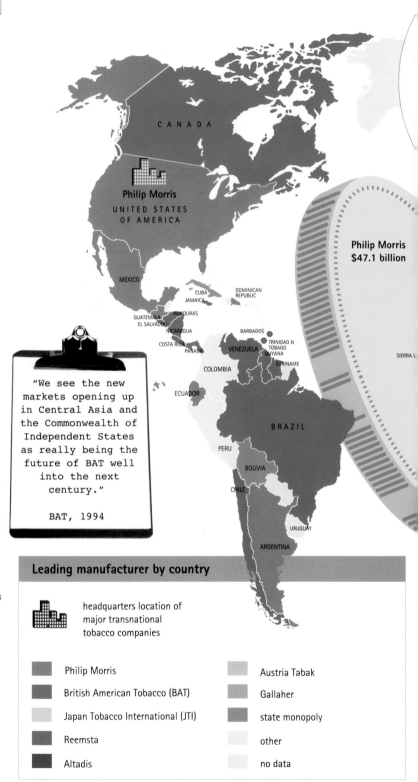

Philip Morris

UNITED STATES
OF AMERICA

Philip Morris
$47.1 billion

"We see the new markets opening up in Central Asia and the Commonwealth of Independent States as really being the future of BAT well into the next century."

BAT, 1994

Leading manufacturer by country

headquarters location of major transnational tobacco companies

- Philip Morris
- British American Tobacco (BAT)
- Japan Tobacco International (JTI)
- Reemsta
- Altadis
- Austria Tabak
- Gallaher
- state monopoly
- other
- no data

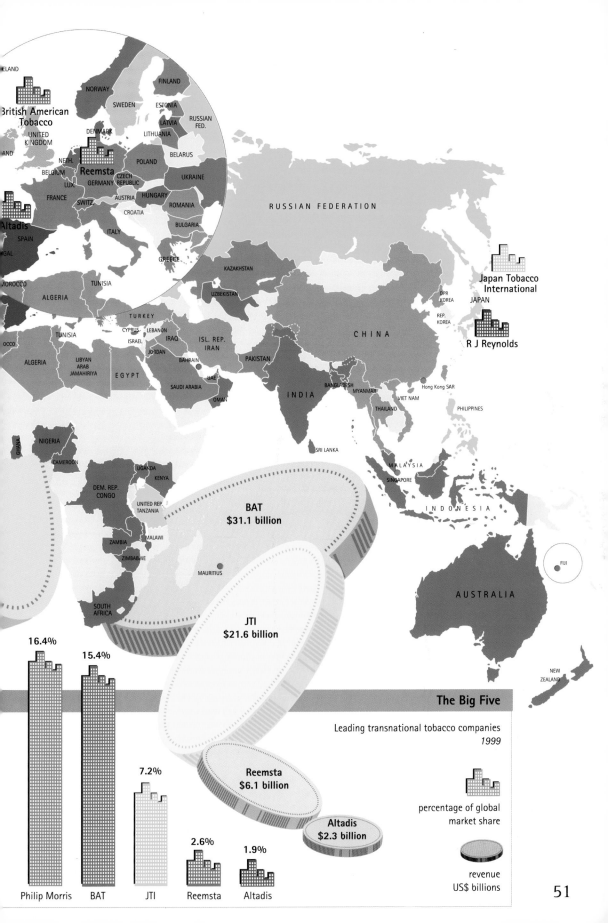

British American
Tobacco
UNITED
KINGDOM

Reemsta

Altadis

Japan Tobacco
International

R J Reynolds

BAT
$31.1 billion

JTI
$21.6 billion

Reemsta
$6.1 billion

Altadis
$2.3 billion

The Big Five

Leading transnational tobacco companies
1999

percentage of global
market share

revenue
US$ billions

16.4%

15.4%

7.2%

2.6%

1.9%

Philip Morris   BAT   JTI   Reemsta   Altadis

51

Tobacco Trade

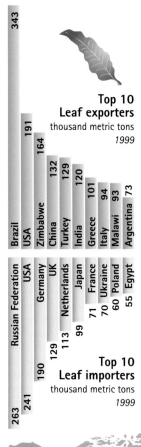

Top 10 Leaf exporters
thousand metric tons
1999

343 Brazil
191 USA
164 Zimbabwe
132 China
129 Turkey
120 India
101 Greece
94 Italy
93 Malawi
73 Argentina

Top 10 Leaf importers
thousand metric tons
1999

263 Russian Federation
241 USA
190 Germany
129 UK
113 Netherlands
99 Japan
71 France
70 Ukraine
60 Poland
55 Egypt

Tobacco trade is big business, for both the raw material (tobacco leaves) and the finished product (manufactured cigarettes).

Brazil is the largest exporter of tobacco leaf, and the Russian Federation and the USA are the largest importers. Some countries that grow tobacco, such as the USA, also import foreign tobacco as well as exporting their own tobacco leaves. Interestingly, the USA exports approximately the same amount of tobacco that it imports. Because US tobacco is popular globally, and tends to be more expensive than tobacco from other countries, the value of US tobacco leaf exports are about double that of the same quantity of imports.

Manufactured cigarettes are also traded globally. Again, the USA is the largest exporter of manufactured cigarettes, accounting for nearly 20 percent of the world total. Japan is the largest importer of cigarettes.

According to government reports, 846 billion cigarettes were exported, but only 619 billion were reported to be imported. Statistics such as these provide a sense of the size of the cigarette smuggling problem.

China is quietly emerging as a significant cigarette exporter, increasing from virtually no exports in 1980 to over 20 billion cigarettes exported in 2001, worth about US$320 million. In 2005 the value of China's export trade in cigarettes is predicted to be US$600 million.

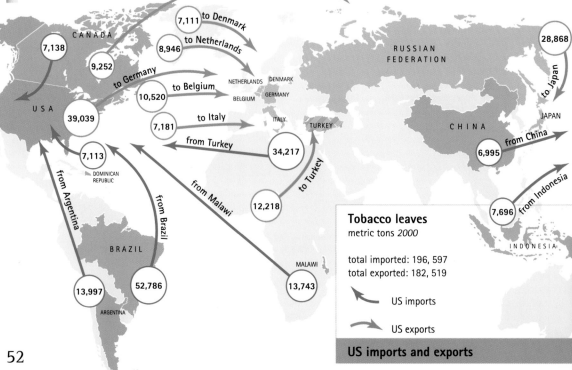

Tobacco leaves
metric tons *2000*

total imported: 196, 597
total exported: 182, 519

↖ US imports

↗ US exports

US imports and exports

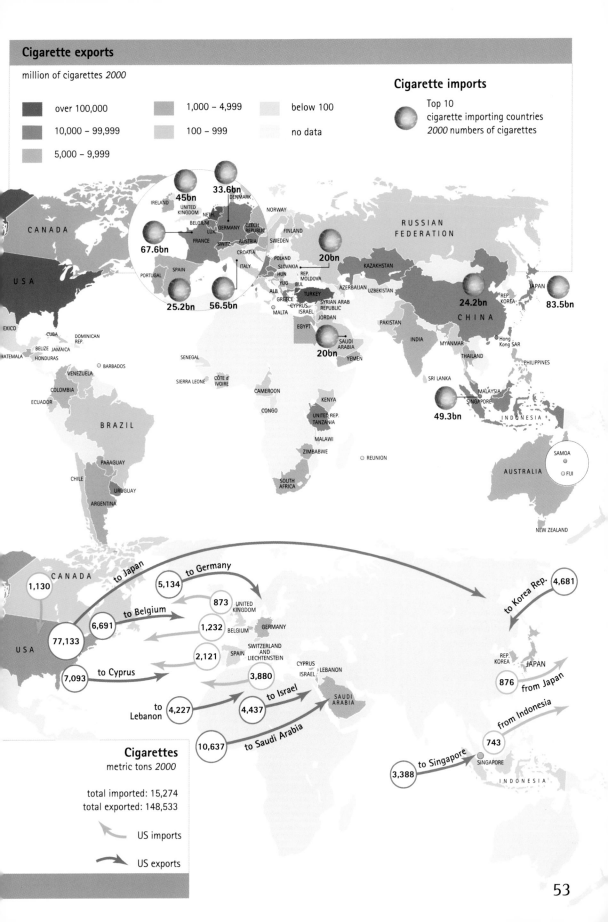

16 | Smuggling

"...price is only one of many factors that influence smuggling rates. Other more important factors include: the tobacco industry's own role in facilitating smuggling; the lack of appropriate controls on tobacco products in international trade; and the existence of entrenched smuggling networks, unlicensed distribution, lax anti-smuggling laws, weak enforcement and official corruption." WHO, 2000

Between 300 and 400 billion cigarettes were smuggled in 1995, equal to about one third of all the legally imported cigarettes.

Cigarettes are the world's most widely smuggled legal consumer product. They are smuggled across almost every national border by constantly changing routes.

Cigarette smuggling causes immeasurable harm. International brands become affordable to low-income consumers and to image-conscious young people in developing countries. Illegal cigarettes evade legal restrictions and health regulations, and while the tobacco companies reap their profits, governments lose tax revenue.

Some governments are now suing tobacco companies for revenue lost due to smuggling activities allegedly condoned by the companies. Measures needed to control smuggling should include monitoring cigarette routes, using technologically sophisticated tax-paid markings on tobacco products, printing unique serial numbers on all packages of tobacco products, and increasing penalties.

CANADA

UNITED STATES OF AMERICA

Montréal

ST. MAARTEN

Aruba

PANAMA   VENEZUELA   GUYANA

COLOMBIA

ECUADOR

BRAZIL

PERU

Iquique

PARAGUAY

Encarnación

CHILE

ARGENTINA

Projected share if no action taken

36% 2003-04

34% 2002-03

32% **2001-02**

25% 2000-01

21% 2000-01

22% 2001-02

21% 2002-03

20% 2003-04

18% 1999-2000

Projected share if new measures are taken and duty increased by 5%

12% 1998-99

6% 1997-98

4% 1996-97

Tackling tobacco smuggling
Cigarettes smuggled into the UK as percentage of market share
1996 – 2004 projected

Lost revenue
Tax revenue lost for each lorry load smuggled into the European Union US$ *1997*

Live animals $24,000

Milk powder $36,000

54

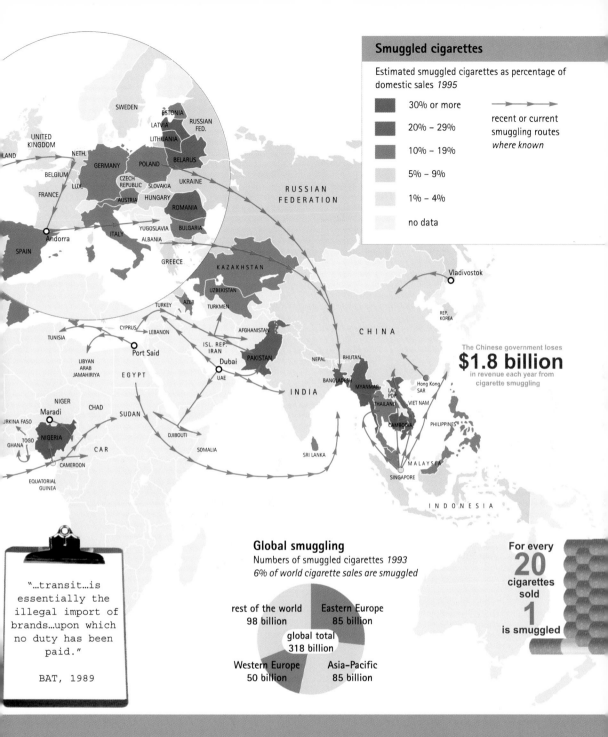

Smuggled cigarettes

Estimated smuggled cigarettes as percentage of domestic sales *1995*

- 30% or more
- 20% – 29%
- 10% – 19%
- 5% – 9%
- 1% – 4%
- no data

→ recent or current smuggling routes *where known*

The Chinese government loses

$1.8 billion

in revenue each year from cigarette smuggling

"…transit…is essentially the illegal import of brands…upon which no duty has been paid."

BAT, 1989

Global smuggling

Numbers of smuggled cigarettes *1993*
6% of world cigarette sales are smuggled

rest of the world
98 billion

Eastern Europe
85 billion

global total
318 billion

Western Europe
50 billion

Asia-Pacific
85 billion

For every

20
cigarettes sold

1
is smuggled

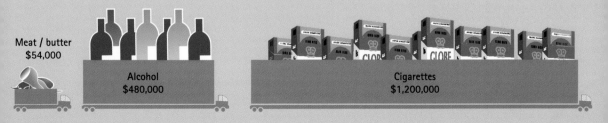

Meat / butter
$54,000

Alcohol
$480,000

Cigarettes
$1,200,000

55

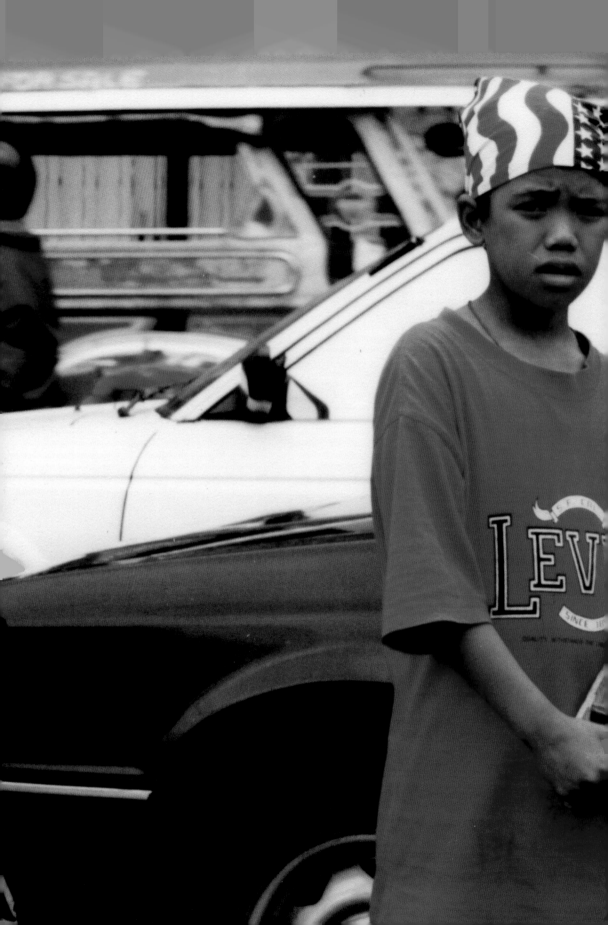

PART 4

PROMOTION

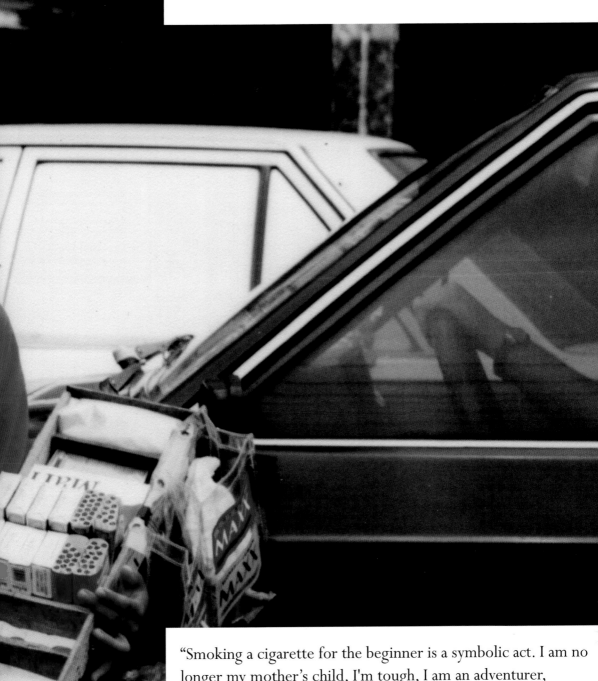

Tom Osdene,
"Why one smokes",
quoted in *How Do You Sell Death*,
Campaign for Tobacco Free Kids,
Washington DC, 2001

"Smoking a cigarette for the beginner is a symbolic act. I am no longer my mother's child, I'm tough, I am an adventurer, I'm not square. Whatever the individual talent, the act of smoking remains a symbolic declaration of personal identity... As the force from the psychological symbolism subsides, the pharmacological effect takes over to sustain the habit."

Cigarettes are possibly the most marketed product in the world. While there is no reliable estimate of global cigarette marketing expenditures, it is clearly in the tens of billions of US dollars a year.

In the USA alone over $10 billion is spent a year on marketing cigarettes, and this at a time when advertising is prohibited on television and radio, when there are limitations on certain types of outdoor advertising and sponsorship, and when cigarette sales are falling. Annual marketing expenditure is over $200 per smoker, and over 46 cents for every pack sold. Promotional allowances, that is payments made to retailers to facilitate sales, account for 41 percent of the total expenditure on cigarette marketing.

Cigarette marketing is bolder and more aggressive in developing countries than it is in the developed world. Cigarette advertising on television and radio is common, and a variety of other venues are exploited. These include sports, arts, pop, fashion and street events, adventure tours, contests, give-aways and the internet.

There are also the hidden advertisements such as the placement of cigarette smoking and tobacco products in films. In addition there is sponsorship of universities, good-will donations for community events, and advertising of other goods and products bearing the cigarette name. Such marketing is seen throughout both the developed and the developing world.

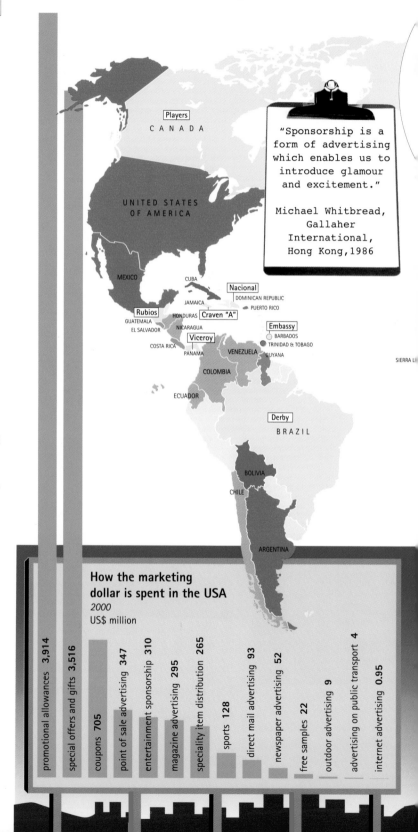

"Sponsorship is a form of advertising which enables us to introduce glamour and excitement."

Michael Whitbread, Gallaher International, Hong Kong, 1986

How the marketing dollar is spent in the USA
2000
US$ million

category	US$ million
promotional allowances	3,914
special offers and gifts	3,516
coupons	705
point of sale advertising	347
entertainment sponsorship	310
magazine advertising	295
speciality item distribution	265
sports	128
direct mail advertising	93
newspaper advertising	52
free samples	22
outdoor advertising	9
advertising on public transport	4
internet advertising	0.95

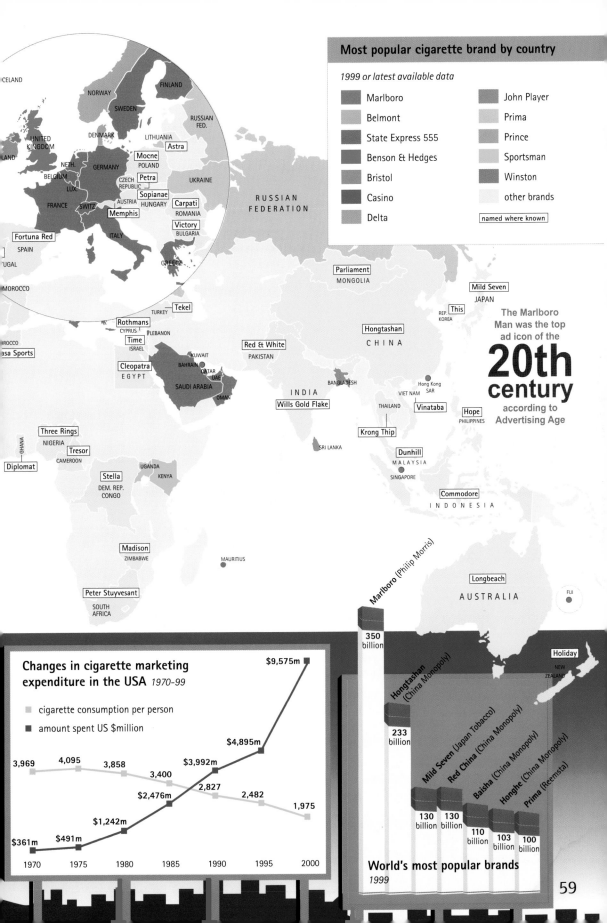

Most popular cigarette brand by country

1999 or latest available data

- Marlboro
- Belmont
- State Express 555
- Benson & Hedges
- Bristol
- Casino
- Delta
- John Player
- Prima
- Prince
- Sportsman
- Winston
- other brands

named where known

Map labels:

ICELAND · NORWAY · SWEDEN · FINLAND · RUSSIAN FED. · DENMARK · LITHUANIA · UNITED KINGDOM · NETH. · BELGIUM · GERMANY · POLAND · UKRAINE · LUX. · FRANCE · SWITZ. · AUSTRIA · HUNGARY · CZECH REPUBLIC · ROMANIA · BULGARIA · ITALY · GREECE · TURKEY · CYPRUS · LEBANON · ISRAEL · SPAIN · PORTUGAL · MOROCCO

Astra · Mocne · Petra · Sopianae · Memphis · Carpati · Victory · Fortuna Red · Tekel · Rothmans · Time · Cleopatra (EGYPT)

Parliament MONGOLIA
Mild Seven JAPAN
This REP. KOREA
Hongtashan CHINA
Red & White PAKISTAN
Wills Gold Flake INDIA
Hong Kong SAR
VIET NAM · Vinataba
THAILAND
Hope PHILIPPINES
Krong Thip
Dunhill MALAYSIA
SINGAPORE
Commodore INDONESIA

KUWAIT · BAHRAIN · QATAR · UAE · SAUDI ARABIA · OMAN · BANGLADESH · SRI LANKA

Three Rings NIGERIA
Tresor CAMEROON
Diplomat
GHANA
Stella DEM. REP. CONGO
UGANDA · KENYA
Madison ZIMBABWE
MAURITIUS
Peter Stuyvesant SOUTH AFRICA

Longbeach AUSTRALIA
Holiday NEW ZEALAND
FIJI

The Marlboro Man was the top ad icon of the

20th century

according to Advertising Age

Changes in cigarette marketing expenditure in the USA *1970-99*

- cigarette consumption per person
- amount spent US $million

Year	consumption per person	amount spent US $million
1970	3,969	$361m
1975	4,095	$491m
1980	3,858	$1,242m
1985	3,400	$2,476m
1990	2,827	$3,992m
		$4,895m
1995	2,482	
2000	1,975	$9,575m

World's most popular brands
1999

- Marlboro (Philip Morris) — 350 billion
- Hongtashan (China Monopoly) — 233 billion
- Mild Seven (Japan Tobacco) — 130 billion
- Red China (China Monopoly) — 130 billion
- Baisha (China Monopoly) — 110 billion
- Honghe (China Monopoly) — 103 billion
- Prima (Reemtsa) — 100 billion

Internet Sales

"The ideal product to sell online would be easy to pack and ship, be much cheaper than what's charged at the retail counter, and be craved by tens of millions of people every day. Cigarettes, the internet was made for you."
David Streitfeld, *Washington Post*, 2000

Cigarette vendors are very easy to locate online by the simplest search mechanisms.

This mode of purchase translates into global penetration of tobacco products, unprecedented access of cigarettes to minors, cheap cigarettes through tax avoidance and smuggling, and unfettered advertising, marketing and promotion.

It is often impossible to identify the country of origin of such vendors. The majority appear to be in Europe and the USA, but countries as varied as Cyprus and Panama also offer internet sales. Strangely, some vendors take credit card details from prospective purchasers but then neither charge nor dispatch any cigarettes.

The internet is also used by tobacco interests to undertake sophisticated public relations, to denigrate pro-health organisations and individuals, to undermine the science of tobacco, and to attack tobacco control legislation (see map 20). Legislation has not yet caught up with this new threat to health.

Sales of cigarettes and other forms of tobacco over the internet started in earnest in the mid-1990s, and are predicted to rise in future.

WHERE ARE THE GOODS?

Test ordering from **12** websites which claim to offer low price cigarettes to the UK market *2001*

3 sites sent cigarettes

1 site charged but did not send cigarettes

8 sites took no money and sent no cigarettes

Prices quoted for 200 cigarettes   **£10 – £27**

Retail price in UK   **£38.60**

Price in UK if intercepted by Customs   **£38.15**

"Most sites offering cheap cigarettes are a rip off. All cigarettes bought via the Internet must bear UK taxes. There are no allowances or loopholes. Cigarettes bought from sites that do not arrange payment of UK taxes are liable to forfeiture. In the last year Customs have destroyed over 10 million such cigarettes."

HM Customs and Excise, UK *2000*

"Philip Morris admits being behind Wavesnet website, an internet company set up to run fashion parades and rave parties where cigarettes are sold at a discount."

Australian Associated Press, *2000*

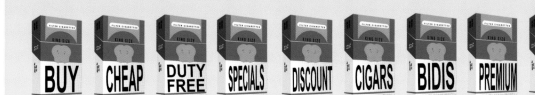

BUY CHEAP DUTY FREE SPECIALS DISCOUNT CIGARS BIDIS PREMIUM TOBACCO

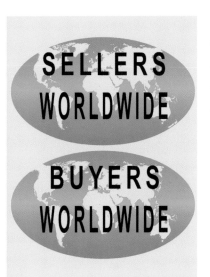

SELLERS WORLDWIDE

BUYERS WORLDWIDE

INTERNET CIGARETTE SEARCH   Google, 2002

Search term	Results found
discount cigarette	9,070
cheap cigarette	5,510
tax free cigarette	1,540
mail order cigarette	374

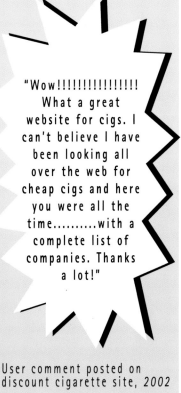

"Wow!!!!!!!!!!!!!!!!! What a great website for cigs. I can't believe I have been looking all over the web for cheap cigs and here you were all the time.........with a complete list of companies. Thanks a lot!"

User comment posted on discount cigarette site, 2002

INTERNET CIGARETTE VENDORS, USA 2000

internet cigarette vendor sites	88
sites with Surgeon-General's warning	24%
sites selling bidis	8%
sites with special promotions	33%
sites with age warning	81%
types of age verification required:	
customer self-reporting they are over 18	49%
typing in a birth date	15%
entering driving license information	9%
US teenagers with internet access	over 50%

The tobacco industry spends millions of dollars trying to influence public policy. It makes major contributions to elected officials and political parties, payments to governments to support infrastructure such as mass transit and large investments in sophisticated public relations campaigns. The industry also gives money to civic, educational and charitable organisations and a host of others.

Since 1995 US tobacco companies have donated more than $32 million in political contributions to state and federal candidates and political parties in the USA, with over 80 percent of this paid to influence federal elections and officeholders. From 1995 to 2000 current members of the US Congress have received over $5 million in contributions from tobacco companies, and nearly six out of ten have accepted tobacco money.

The tobacco industry sought to delay, and eventually defeat, the EC directive on tobacco advertising and sponsorship by seeking the aid of figures at the highest levels of European politics while at times attempting to conceal the industry's role. Parliamentarians in Europe have accepted money and even senior positions in tobacco companies.

Tobacco companies also attempt to influence the political process, by subsidising the air travel of candidates and their staff, funding political conventions and inaugurations, and hosting fundraisers. As well as campaign contributions, tobacco companies conduct direct lobbying and sophisticated public relations campaigns, including paid media, to influence the opinions of political decision-makers.

Comprehensive tobacco legislation was defeated in the US Senate in 1998. Those who voted against the legislation had received on average, nearly four times as much money from the tobacco industry in the two years before their last election, as those who voted in favour of the bill.

Buying influence and favours through political contributions is common practice; however, most countries do not require mandatory reporting.

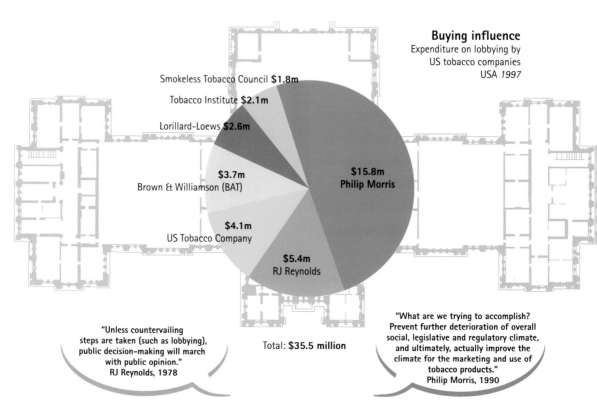

Buying influence
Expenditure on lobbying by US tobacco companies
USA *1997*

Smokeless Tobacco Council **$1.8m**

Tobacco Institute **$2.1m**

Lorillard-Loews **$2.6m**

$3.7m
Brown & Williamson (BAT)

$4.1m
US Tobacco Company

$15.8m
Philip Morris

$5.4m
RJ Reynolds

Total: **$35.5 million**

"Unless countervailing steps are taken (such as lobbying), public decision-making will march with public opinion."
RJ Reynolds, 1978

"What are we trying to accomplish? Prevent further deterioration of overall social, legislative and regulatory climate, and ultimately, actually improve the climate for the marketing and use of tobacco products."
Philip Morris, 1990

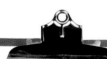

"Small shopkeepers were enlisted to write protests to members of Parliament; the letters 'some with deliberate typographical errors to create the aura of authenticity,' were prepared by the (tobacco) industry for the shopkeepers."

Philip Morris, 1990

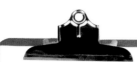

"We have got the unions to support industry in several countries. Prominent have been the efforts they have made on the tax issues in the UK where they were very involved in a letter writing campaign to Members of Parliament."

Philip Morris, 1985

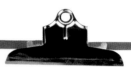

"Philip Morris and the industry are positively impacting the government decisions of Bahrain, Kuwait, Oman, Qatar, Saudi Arabia and the UAE through the creative use of market specific studies, position papers, well briefed distributors who lobby, media owners and consultants…"

Philip Morris, 1987

"Turning now to primary and passive smoking…To get more favorable press, we are contemplating organizing another journalists' conference similar to the one we put together in Madrid for Latin American journalists in 1984."

Philip Morris, 1985

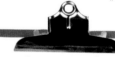

"The International Tobacco Growers Association could 'front' for our third world lobby activities at WHO, and gain support from nations hostile to multinational corporations…"

INFOTAB,
(tobacco industry pressure group), 1988

Buying favours
Top tobacco contributions to federal candidates
USA *1995–2000*

- Philip Morris $10.2m
- RJ Reynolds $4.7m
- $3.4m US Tobacco Company
- $2.9m Brown and Williamson (BAT)
- $1.2m Tobacco Institute
- $0.6 Lorillard Tobacco
- $0.6m Smokeless Tobacco Council
- $0.4 Swisher International
- $0.3m Conwood Company
- $0.2m Pinkerton Tobacco Company

Smokers' Rights Organisations

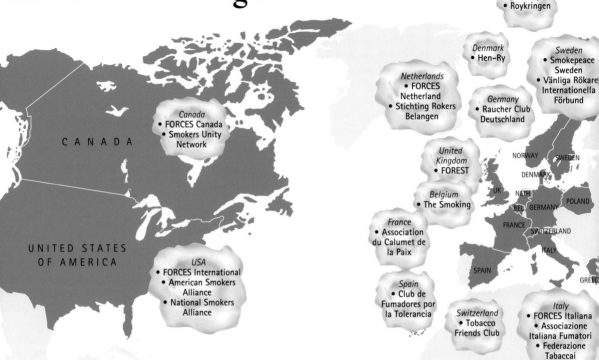

Norway
• Roykringen

Denmark
• Hen–Ry

Sweden
• Smokepeace Sweden
• Vänliga Rökare Internationella Förbund

Netherlands
• FORCES Netherland
• Stichting Rokers Belangen

Germany
• Raucher Club Deutschland

Canada
• FORCES Canada
• Smokers Unity Network

United Kingdom
• FOREST

Belgium
• The Smoking

France
• Association du Calumet de la Paix

USA
• FORCES International
• American Smokers Alliance
• National Smokers Alliance

Spain
• Club de Fumadores por la Tolerancia

Switzerland
• Tobacco Friends Club

Italy
• FORCES Italiana
• Associazione Italiana Fumatori
• Federazione Tabaccai

CANADA

UNITED STATES OF AMERICA

NORWAY SWEDEN DENMARK UK NETH BEL GERMANY POLAND FRANCE SWITZERLAND ITALY SPAIN GREEC

The tobacco industry has long appreciated the importance and difficulty of mobilising smokers to speak out on behalf of smokers' rights. Consequently the tobacco companies have investigated ways that they could "stimulate" the development of groups of smokers, so as to have the support, or at least the appearance of support from smokers and other "natural or third party allies".

There are fewer than two dozen smokers' rights organisations in the world, and all are in the developed world. The tobacco industry documents illustrate that while many of these organisations purport to be independent of the tobacco industry, at least some are dependent on tobacco company funding. In a 1988 document, the head of Philip Morris said, "Should we strive to set up FOREST type organisations throughout our regions?".

At the request of Philip Morris the public relations firm of Burson-Marstellar formed the National Smokers Alliance, a smokers rights group, in 1993. Philip Morris initially provided the National Smokers Alliance with $4 million in seed funding. Documents show that Philip Morris formed similar groups throughout Europe. These "grassroots" groups, with their facades of "independence" from the industry, allowed them to do and say things publicly that tobacco companies could not.

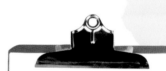

"To sum up, then, on using our natural allies. We have made a start; we have proved that it can be done; we have found that they can be a very effective force; and we intend to do more in the future."

Philip Morris, 1985

Smokers' Rights Organisations

2002 where known

FOREST: Freedom Organisation for the Right
to Enjoy Smoking Tobacco

FORCES: Fight Ordinances & Restrictions
to Control & Eliminate Smoking

Russian Federation
• FORCES International

RUSSIAN FEDERATION

Poland
Towarzystwo Ochrony Palacych

Greece
• Eleftheria

"Smokers are not a constituency that can be easily rallied. They are defensive, often self-deprecating, somewhat shamed. May see themselves engaged in a habit they wish they could quit. They are a passive group. Expressing very little anger or resentment. There is no sign among them of any significant determination to assert their rights as smokers."

RJ Reynolds, 1978

"We try to keep Philip Morris out of media issues like taxation, smoking bans and marketing restrictions. Instead, we try to provide the media with statements in support of our positions from third party sources, which carry more credibility than our company and have no apparent vested interest."

Philip Morris, 1993

"First we must work harder at getting smokers to help the industry. If we are to have any success at changing the climate of opinion, we have to get the smokers more on our side, or at least enough of them to start to make a difference."

Philip Morris, 1985

"In Australia too, through FOREST, we have awakened the public in the tax area, with carefully orchestrated campaigns."

Philip Morris, 1985

AUSTRALIA

New Zealand
• FORCES New Zealand
• Smokers of the World Unite

NEW ZEALAND

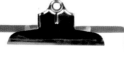
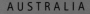

"On May 12, 1994, an unsolicited box of what appeared to be tobacco company documents was delivered to Professor Stanton Glantz...The documents in the box dated from the early 1950's to the early 1980's. They consisted primarily of confidential internal memoranda related to B&W and BAT. Many of the documents contained internal discussions of the tobacco industry's public relations and legal strategies over the years, and they were often labelled "confidential" or 'privileged.' The return address on the box was simply 'Mr Butts'."

So starts *The Cigarette Papers*, the first report chronicling the release of previously secret tobacco industry documents. Public release of these documents clearly illustrated their power in exposing tobacco industry corporate behaviour, and they profoundly influenced public opinion.

Following the release of the BAT documents and as a result of litigation and legal settlement agreements in the USA, documents introduced through legal discovery have had to be made publicly available by the tobacco industry in physical depositories in Minneapolis, USA and Guildford, UK.

As a result of the 1998 Master Settlement Agreement between 46 states and the tobacco industry, the documents of the Minnesota Depository are to be duplicated online via searchable websites maintained by each of the companies.

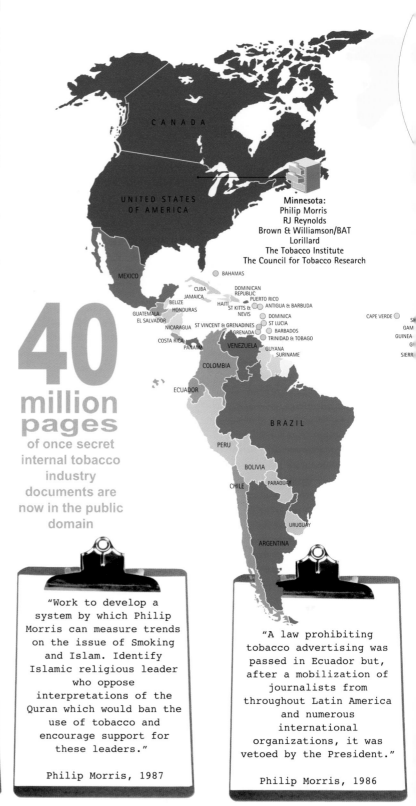

Minnesota:
Philip Morris
RJ Reynolds
Brown & Williamson/BAT
Lorillard
The Tobacco Institute
The Council for Tobacco Research

40 million pages of once secret internal tobacco industry documents are now in the public domain

"Our work in Senegal resulted in a new advertising decree which reversed a total advertising ban."

Philip Morris, 1986

"Work to develop a system by which Philip Morris can measure trends on the issue of Smoking and Islam. Identify Islamic religious leader who oppose interpretations of the Quran which would ban the use of tobacco and encourage support for these leaders."

Philip Morris, 1987

"A law prohibiting tobacco advertising was passed in Ecuador but, after a mobilization of journalists from throughout Latin America and numerous international organizations, it was vetoed by the President."

Philip Morris, 1986

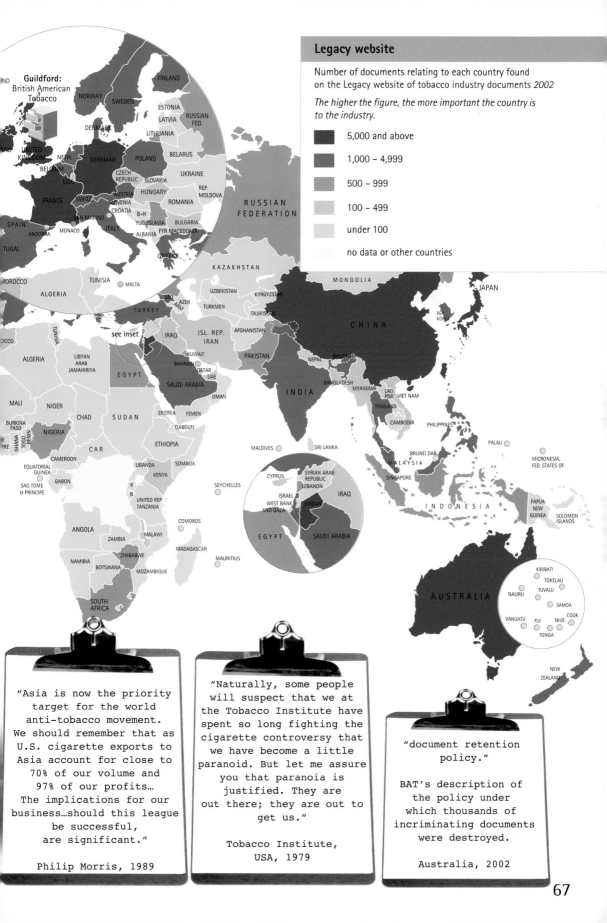

Legacy website

Number of documents relating to each country found on the Legacy website of tobacco industry documents *2002*

The higher the figure, the more important the country is to the industry.

- 5,000 and above
- 1,000 – 4,999
- 500 – 999
- 100 – 499
- under 100
- no data or other countries

Guildford: British American Tobacco

see inset

> "Asia is now the priority target for the world anti-tobacco movement. We should remember that as U.S. cigarette exports to Asia account for close to 70% of our volume and 97% of our profits... The implications for our business...should this league be successful, are significant."
>
> Philip Morris, 1989

> "Naturally, some people will suspect that we at the Tobacco Institute have spent so long fighting the cigarette controversy that we have become a little paranoid. But let me assure you that paranoia is justified. They are out there; they are out to get us."
>
> Tobacco Institute, USA, 1979

> "document retention policy."
>
> BAT's description of the policy under which thousands of incriminating documents were destroyed.
>
> Australia, 2002

67

PART 5

TAKING ACTION

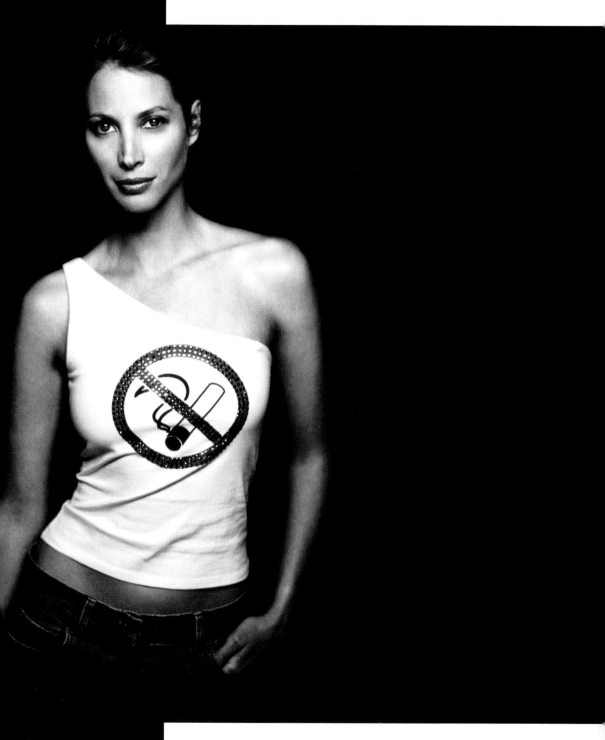

"One never notices what has been done; one can only see what remains to be done."

Marie Curie (1867-1934)

Basic scientific epidemiological research over the last 50 years has proved the harmfulness of tobacco.

Reducing tobacco use requires knowing what works, and applying this information systematically. Building the scientific base is a prerequisite for progress. In developed countries, there has been no shortage of data on tobacco use. Thanks in part to investments by international development agencies and foundations, tobacco control research in the developing world is also beginning to flourish.

While increased funding is important, barriers continue to exist. A recent report highlighted recurring research themes for developing countries, including the lack of standardised data, absence of a network for communication, lack of tobacco control research capacity, and the need for human and financial resources.

The source of the funding is of equal importance. Historically, tobacco companies have sponsored research, promising complete independence, only to bury unfavourable findings and delete words such as "cancer." To improve their public image, tobacco companies are once again offering substantial research funding to academic institutions worldwide, promising complete independence. Academic researchers should consider this option cautiously, given the history of misuse of scientific findings.

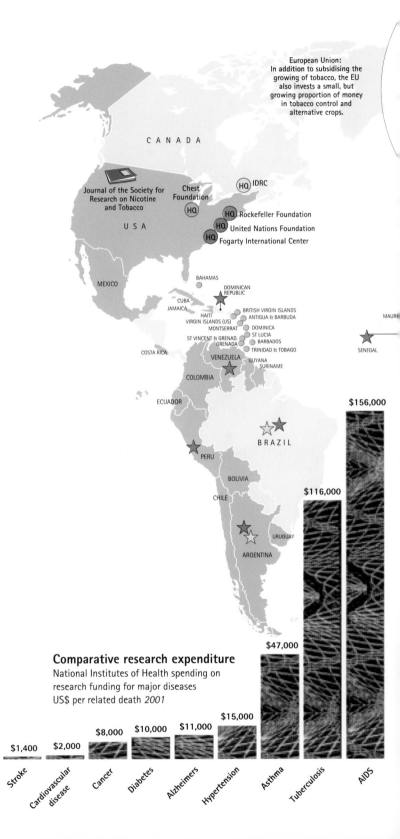

Comparative research expenditure
National Institutes of Health spending on research funding for major diseases
US$ per related death *2001*

Tobacco use	$1,000
Stroke	$1,400
Cardiovascular disease	$2,000
Cancer	$8,000
Diabetes	$10,000
Alzheimers	$11,000
Hypertension	$15,000
Asthma	$47,000
Tuberculosis	$116,000
AIDS	$156,000

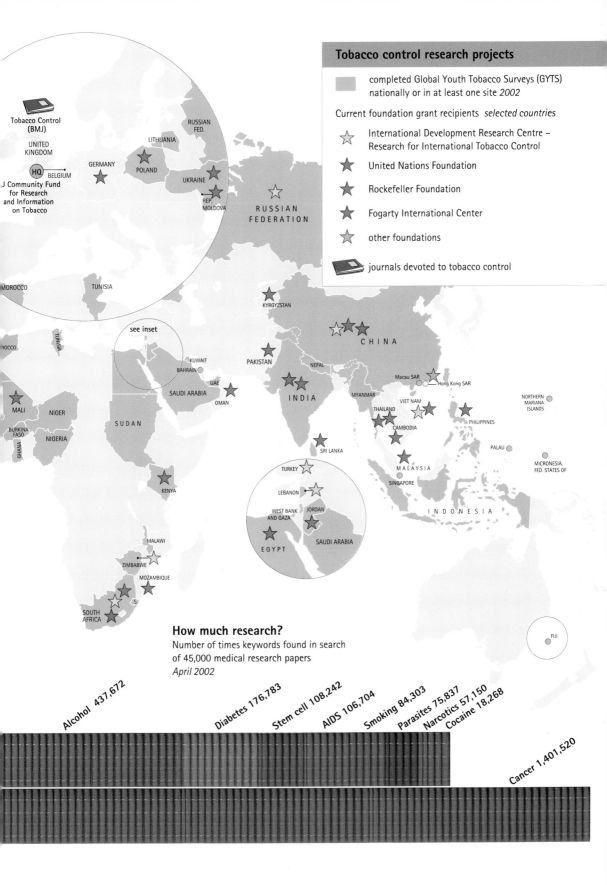

Tobacco control research projects

completed Global Youth Tobacco Surveys (GYTS) nationally or in at least one site *2002*

Current foundation grant recipients *selected countries*

International Development Research Centre – Research for International Tobacco Control

United Nations Foundation

Rockefeller Foundation

Fogarty International Center

other foundations

journals devoted to tobacco control

Tobacco Control (BMJ)
UNITED KINGDOM

HQ BELGIUM

J Community Fund for Research and Information on Tobacco

see inset

How much research?
Number of times keywords found in search of 45,000 medical research papers
April 2002

Alcohol 437,672   Diabetes 176,783   Stem cell 108,242   AIDS 106,704   Smoking 84,303   Parasites 75,837   Narcotics 57,150   Cocaine 18,268

Cancer 1,401,520

71

Tobacco Control Organisations

The tobacco control network is committed and far-reaching. The World Health Organization's Tobacco Free Initiative (TFI) is conducted from headquarters in Geneva and the regional and national offices around the world. There is now a WHO Focal Point on Tobacco or Health in all countries, and the TFI is supported by a number of other international agencies such as Unicef, the World Bank, IARC and the UN Foundation.

The non-governmental organisations (NGOs) highlighted on this map are those whose remit is 100 percent tobacco-related. There are dozens more international NGOs which address tobacco control as part of their activities, ranging from the World Medical Association to Consumers International. Academia is also a valuable partner, as many universities carry out research and promote policy initiatives in tobacco control.

There are also many national tobacco control organisations whose impact is not restricted to that country but also felt worldwide. These include ASH in the UK, ThaiHealth in Thailand, and the Campaign for Tobacco Free Kids in the USA. In addition, many national NGOs work part time on tobacco issues. Numerous other partners include organisations involved with women, youth, environment, law, economics, human rights, religion and development.

Most tobacco control organisations are seriously under-funded given the scope of the tobacco epidemic. The better financed, such as ThaiHealth, are funded by a percentage of tobacco tax.

Chicago
International Tobacco Evidence Network

Middleton, Wisconsin
Society for Research on Nicotine and Tobacco

Boston
Network for Accountability of Tobacco Transnationals

Washington DC
AMRO/PAHO

Washington DC
Global Partnerships for Tobacco Control

New York
Liaison Office with the UN, UN Ad Hoc Interagency Task Force on Tobacco Control

New York
International Network of Women Against Tobacco

Lima
Latin American Coordinating Committee on Tobacco Control

"We cannot hope to win in a head-on confrontation. Our tactics must be to discover our opponents' weaknesses, attack those particular points, cause as much confusion as possible, and attack somewhere else while their attention is distracted… Surprise is a key element."

Philip Morris, 1978

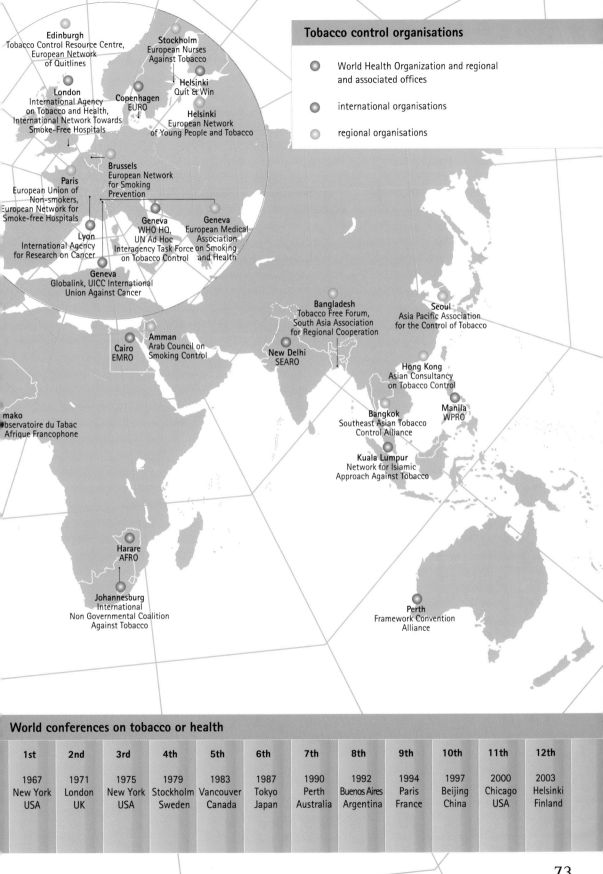

Tobacco control organisations

- World Health Organization and regional and associated offices
- international organisations
- regional organisations

Edinburgh
Tobacco Control Resource Centre,
European Network
of Quitlines

Stockholm
European Nurses
Against Tobacco

Helsinki
Quit & Win

London
International Agency
on Tobacco and Health,
International Network Towards
Smoke-Free Hospitals

Copenhagen
EURO

Helsinki
European Network
of Young People and Tobacco

Brussels
European Network
for Smoking
Prevention

Paris
European Union of
Non-smokers,
European Network for
Smoke-free Hospitals

Geneva
WHO HQ,
UN Ad Hoc
Interagency Task Force on Smoking
on Tobacco Control

Geneva
European Medical
Association
and Health

Lyon
International Agency
for Research on Cancer

Geneva
Globalink, UICC International
Union Against Cancer

Cairo
EMRO

Amman
Arab Council on
Smoking Control

New Delhi
SEARO

Bangladesh
Tobacco Free Forum,
South Asia Association
for Regional Cooperation

Seoul
Asia Pacific Association
for the Control of Tobacco

Hong Kong
Asian Consultancy
on Tobacco Control

mako
Observatoire du Tabac
Afrique Francophone

Bangkok
Southeast Asian Tobacco
Control Alliance

Manila
WPRO

Kuala Lumpur
Network for Islamic
Approach Against Tobacco

Harare
AFRO

Johannesburg
International
Non Governmental Coalition
Against Tobacco

Perth
Framework Convention
Alliance

World conferences on tobacco or health

1st	2nd	3rd	4th	5th	6th	7th	8th	9th	10th	11th	12th
1967 New York USA	1971 London UK	1975 New York USA	1979 Stockholm Sweden	1983 Vancouver Canada	1987 Tokyo Japan	1990 Perth Australia	1992 Buenos Aires Argentina	1994 Paris France	1997 Beijing China	2000 Chicago USA	2003 Helsinki Finland

Banning smoking in public places is a sound public health measure to protect the health of non-smokers.

The issue of workplace bans is primarily one of labour legislation to protect the health of workers, who are exposed to passive smoking for long periods during their work shifts, whether this be in public or office buildings, restaurants or public transport.

Workplace smoking bans are effective in reducing exposure to passive smoking. Smokers who are employed in workplaces with smoking bans are likely to consume fewer cigarettes per day, are more likely to consider quitting, and quit at a greater rate, than smokers employed in workplaces with no or weaker policies.

A total ban works better than a partial ban. Most airlines are now smoke-free and the global trend is towards a safer, cleaner indoor environment in the home and in public and work places.

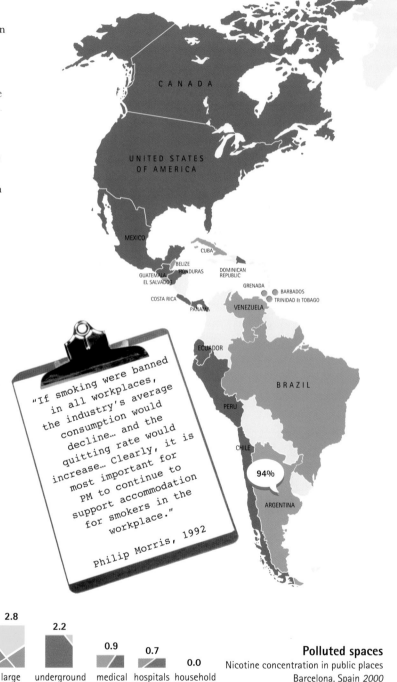

"If smoking were banned in all workplaces, the industry's average consumption would decline... and the quitting rate would increase... Clearly, it is most important for PM to continue to support accommodation for smokers in the workplace."

Philip Morris, 1992

94%

Polluted spaces
Nicotine concentration in public places
Barcelona, Spain *2000*
micrograms per cubic metre

12.4 restaurants
9.5 secondary school
7.9 household smokers
2.8 large stores
2.2 underground subway stations
0.9 medical school
0.7 hospitals
0.0 household non-smoking

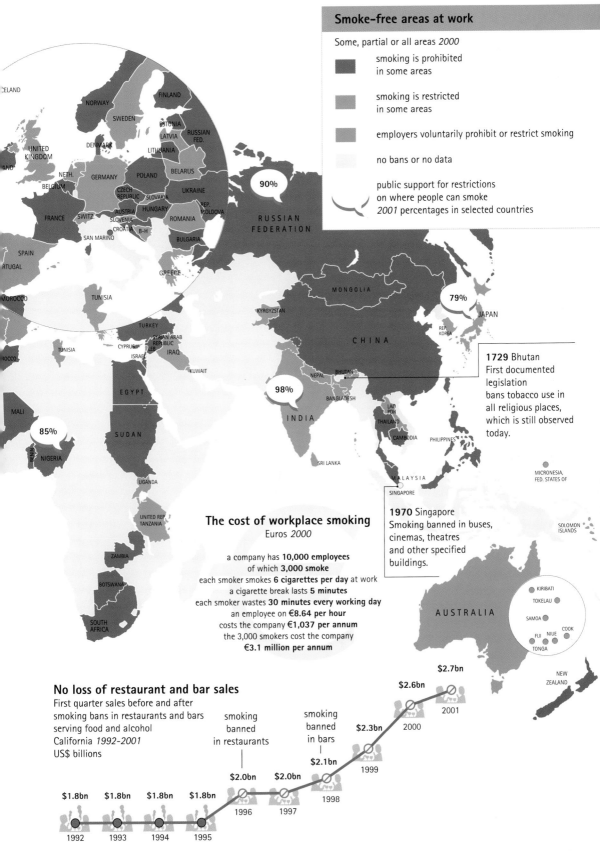

Smoke-free areas at work

Some, partial or all areas *2000*

smoking is prohibited
in some areas

smoking is restricted
in some areas

employers voluntarily prohibit or restrict smoking

no bans or no data

public support for restrictions
on where people can smoke
2001 percentages in selected countries

90%

79%

98%

85%

1729 Bhutan
First documented
legislation
bans tobacco use in
all religious places,
which is still observed
today.

1970 Singapore
Smoking banned in buses,
cinemas, theatres
and other specified
buildings.

The cost of workplace smoking
Euros *2000*

a company has **10,000 employees**
of which **3,000 smoke**
each smoker smokes **6 cigarettes per day** at work
a cigarette break lasts **5 minutes**
each smoker wastes **30 minutes every working day**
an employee on **€8.64 per hour**
costs the company **€1,037 per annum**
the 3,000 smokers cost the company
€3.1 million per annum

No loss of restaurant and bar sales
First quarter sales before and after
smoking bans in restaurants and bars
serving food and alcohol
California *1992-2001*
US$ billions

smoking
banned
in restaurants

smoking
banned
in bars

$2.7bn
2001

$2.6bn
2000

$2.3bn

$2.1bn
1999

$2.0bn
$2.0bn
1998

$1.8bn $1.8bn $1.8bn $1.8bn
1992   1993   1994   1995

1996   1997

Legislation: Advertising Bans

The tobacco industry denies that advertising plays a role in encouraging people to smoke or increasing the amount smoked, but the research suggests otherwise. As governments acknowledge the harm caused by tobacco and the need to discourage its use, restrictions and outright bans on tobacco advertising are becoming common. Partial restrictions are notorious for leading to other forms of marketing supplanting the restriction. Because of the shift of marketing dollars from one medium to another, the evidence suggests that comprehensive bans on all forms of tobacco promotion can be effective in reducing tobacco use, while partial restrictions have limited or no effect.

Cigarette packaging plays an increasingly important role as advertising restrictions are implemented. Packet design plays an important role in establishing brand imagery and competing for potential customers. Many countries are advocating plain packaging. Some also propose the banning of certain words such as "Light" or "Mild" as these may convey the impression that the cigarettes are less harmful or contain fewer harmful constituents.

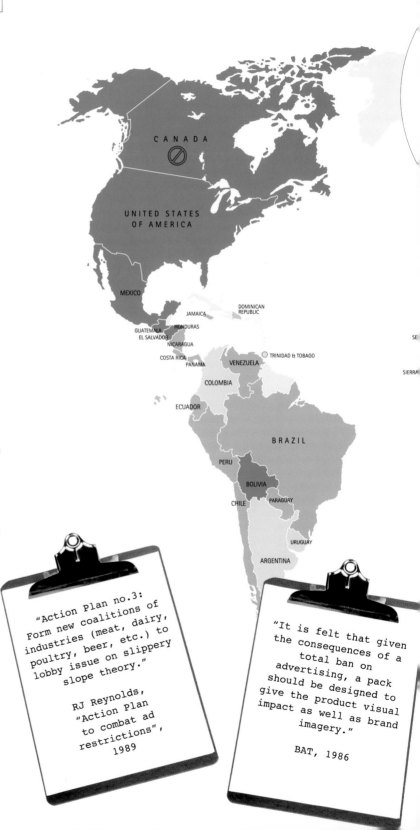

"Action Plan no.3: Form new coalitions of industries (meat, dairy, poultry, beer, etc.) to lobby issue on slippery slope theory."

RJ Reynolds, "Action Plan to combat ad restrictions", 1989

"It is felt that given the consequences of a total ban on advertising, a pack should be designed to give the product visual impact as well as brand imagery."

BAT, 1986

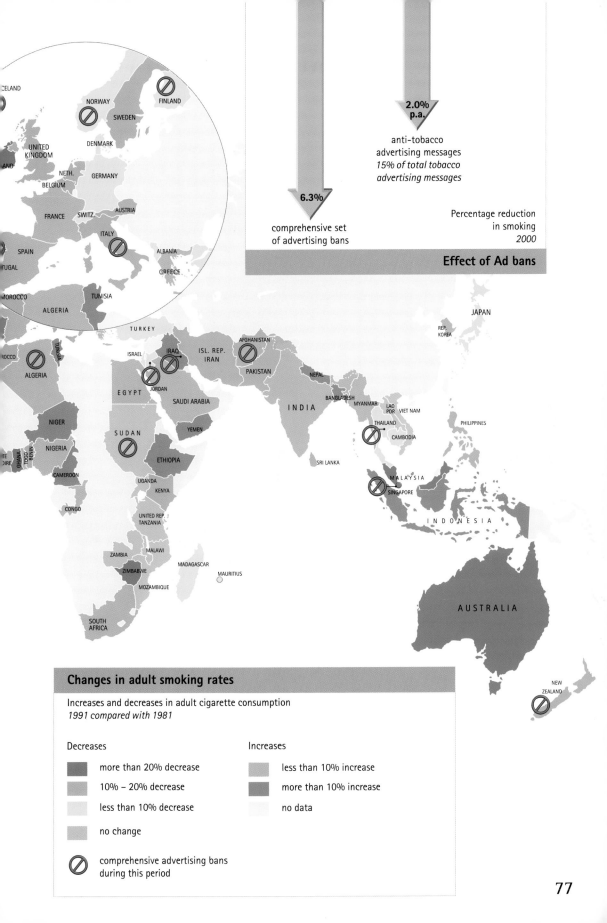

2.0% p.a.

anti-tobacco
advertising messages
*15% of total tobacco
advertising messages*

6.3%

comprehensive set
of advertising bans

Percentage reduction
in smoking
2000

Effect of Ad bans

Changes in adult smoking rates

Increases and decreases in adult cigarette consumption
1991 compared with 1981

Decreases

more than 20% decrease

10% – 20% decrease

less than 10% decrease

no change

comprehensive advertising bans
during this period

Increases

less than 10% increase

more than 10% increase

no data

Legislation: Health Warnings

Health warnings about tobacco have been in existence for four hundred years, starting with King James I in England and Fang Yizhi in China, both in the 17th century (see map 1).

Cigarette packs first carried health warnings in the 1960's following scientific reports on the hazards of smoking in the USA and the UK. These early warnings were weak and inconspicuous. Contemporary Canadian warnings are the most vivid in the world and are serving as the model for other countries, such as Brazil. While many countries have some type of health warning on the pack, these are not universal and many that do exist are not as unequivocal, simple and stark as is necessary; some are not in the local language nor on all tobacco products.

Reports from Canada and Australia suggest that plain packaging may increase both prominence and believability of health warnings. That is, no use of colour, logo or graphic design, but simply a generic pack of cigarettes, with the brand name.

Health authorities now recommend that cigarette packages should not contain tar and nicotine levels as measured by smoking machines, as these do not reflect the actual inhalation of tar and nicotine due to cigarette design (primarily ventilation holes), and individual smoker behaviour (a tendency for

smokers to compensate to get more nicotine from each cigarette) and are thus misleading. Others suggest that a range of values should be presented that better resembles how smokers actually smoke, and

to include this information on the pack of cigarettes in a section on toxic constituents, which also includes levels of carcinogens and carbon monoxide exposure.

"If they reject your pack, they reject your brand."

Brown and Williamson, 2002

GREENLAND

CANADA

UNITED STATES OF AMERICA

BERMUDA

BAHAMAS

MEXICO

CUBA
JAMAICA
BELIZE
HONDURAS
GUATEMALA
EL SALVADOR
NICARAGUA
COSTA RICA
PANAMA

HAITI
DOMINICAN REPUBLIC
ST KITTS &
NEVIS
ST VINCENT & GRENADINES
GRENADA

ANGUILLA
ANTIGUA & BARBUDA
DOMINICA
ST LUCIA
BARBADOS
TRINIDAD & TOBAGO

VENEZUELA
COLOMBIA

GUYANA
SURINAME
FRENCH GUIANA (Fr)

ECUADOR

PERU

BRAZIL

BOLIVIA

CHILE

PARAGUAY

93%

URUGUAY

ARGENTINA

WESTERN SA

MAUR

CAPE VERDE

SI

GAM

GUINEA-
GU

SIERR

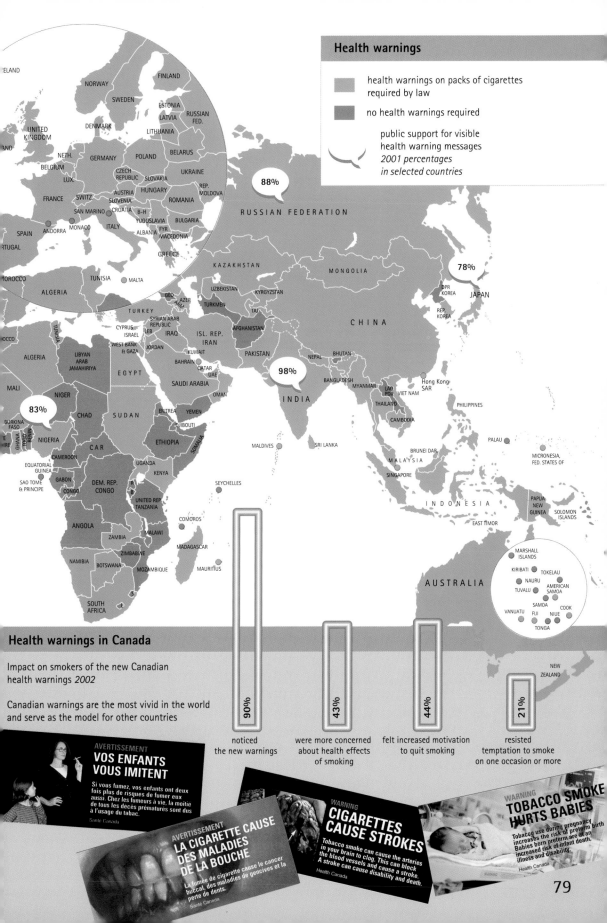

Health warnings

health warnings on packs of cigarettes required by law

no health warnings required

public support for visible health warning messages
2001 percentages in selected countries

88%

78%

98%

83%

Health warnings in Canada

Impact on smokers of the new Canadian health warnings *2002*

Canadian warnings are the most vivid in the world and serve as the model for other countries

90% noticed the new warnings

43% were more concerned about health effects of smoking

44% felt increased motivation to quit smoking

21% resisted temptation to smoke on one occasion or more

AVERTISSEMENT
VOS ENFANTS VOUS IMITENT
Si vous fumez, vos enfants ont deux fois plus de risques de fumer eux aussi. Chez les fumeurs à vie, la moitié de tous les décès prématurés sont dus à l'usage du tabac.
Santé Canada

AVERTISSEMENT
LA CIGARETTE CAUSE DES MALADIES DE LA BOUCHE
La fumée de cigarette cause le cancer buccal, des maladies de gencives et la perte de dents.
Santé Canada

WARNING
CIGARETTES CAUSE STROKES
Tobacco smoke can cause the arteries in your brain to clog. This can block the blood vessels and cause a stroke. A stroke can cause disability and death.
Health Canada

WARNING
TOBACCO SMOKE HURTS BABIES
Tobacco use during pregnancy increases the risk of preterm birth. Babies born preterm are at an increased risk of infant death, illness and disability.
Health Canada

79

Education is essential for sustained progress in tobacco control. Many legislative or tax interventions will not be effective if there is no public understanding, support and demand for such changes. People support tax increases when they understand that the rationale is to reduce youth smoking: an average of 87 percent of respondents in Argentina, India, Japan, Nigeria, and the Russian Federation were in favour of international efforts to create a set of rules and regulations to curb tobacco use.

Schools can provide an ideal venue not only to teach about the harmful effects of smoking, but also to teach students refusal skills and an understanding of the behaviour of the tobacco industry. This includes analysing the manipulation of young people by marketing which equates smoking with growing up, freedom and being cool.

The first step with school programmes is to increase knowledge about the harm caused by smoking and to change beliefs, attitudes and intentions. This alone is not sufficient to change behaviour. A school tobacco control programme must also incorporate prohibiting tobacco use at all school facilities and events, helping students and staff

to quit smoking, and ideally making the course part of a coordinated school health programme, reinforced by community-wide efforts.

To improve its public image, the tobacco industry has recently become active in smoking prevention programmes for young people. These programmes portray smoking as an adult decision, and that young people should wait until they are grown up to decide to smoke. Since young people aspire to be young adults, this type of message may actually make smoking more appealing to youth.

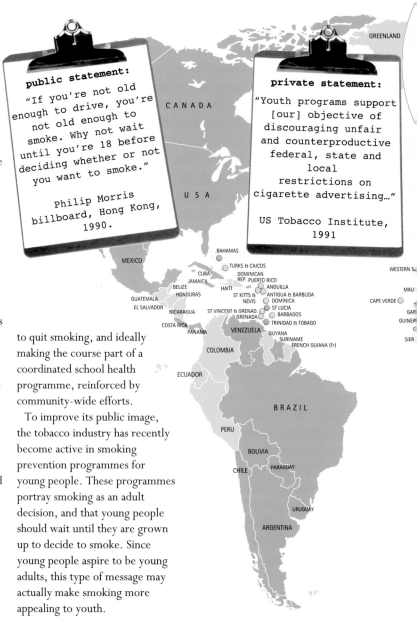

public statement:

"If you're not old enough to drive, you're not old enough to smoke. Why not wait until you're 18 before deciding whether or not you want to smoke."

Philip Morris billboard, Hong Kong, 1990.

private statement:

"Youth programs support [our] objective of discouraging unfair and counterproductive federal, state and local restrictions on cigarette advertising…"

US Tobacco Institute, 1991

World No Tobacco Day: 31st May   annual themes

1988	1989	1990	1991	1992	1993	1994	1995	1996	1997	1998
Tobacco or Health: Choose Health	Women and Tobacco	Growing up without Tobacco	Tobacco in Public Places and on Public Transport	Tobacco at the Workplace	Health Services, including Health Personnel, against Tobacco	The Media against Tobacco	The Economics of Tobacco	Sports and The Arts without Tobacco	The United Nations and Specialized Agencies Against Tobacco "United for a Tobacco-Free World"	Growing up without tobacco

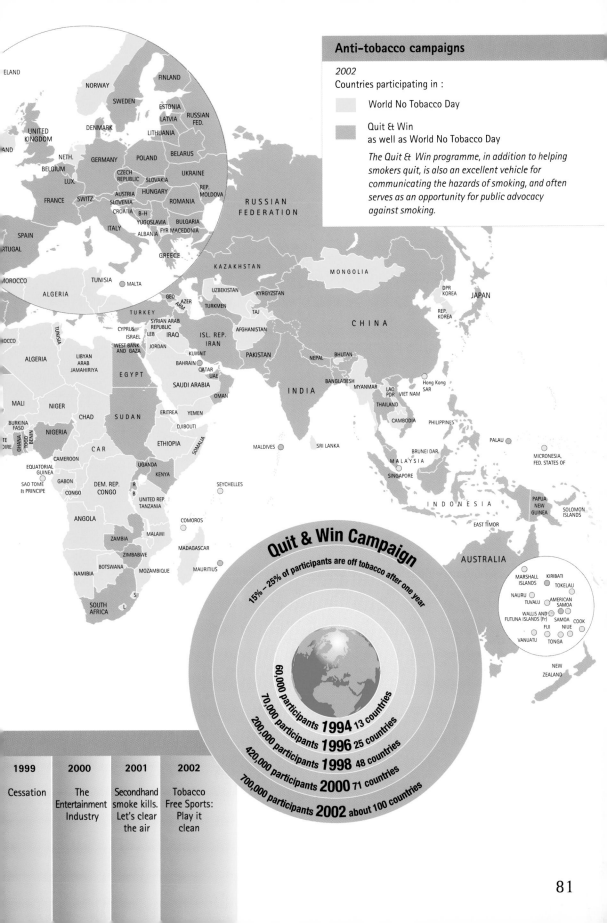

Anti-tobacco campaigns

2002
Countries participating in :

World No Tobacco Day

Quit & Win
as well as World No Tobacco Day

The Quit & Win programme, in addition to helping smokers quit, is also an excellent vehicle for communicating the hazards of smoking, and often serves as an opportunity for public advocacy against smoking.

Quit & Win Campaign

15% – 25% of participants are off tobacco after one year

60,000 participants **1994** 13 countries
70,000 participants **1996** 25 countries
200,000 participants **1998** 48 countries
420,000 participants **2000** 71 countries
700,000 participants **2002** about 100 countries

1999	2000	2001	2002
Cessation	The Entertainment Industry	Secondhand smoke kills. Let's clear the air	Tobacco Free Sports: Play it clean

> "Every nicotine patch sold means 200 cigarettes not sold." Clive Bates, ASH UK, 2002

The main dangers of smoking decrease when smokers quit, even in those who have smoked for 30 or more years.

Smokers move through stages in relation to quitting: of pre-contemplation, contemplation, readiness then action, followed by maintenance or relapse. Many move through this cycle several times before they finally quit, while others report they found it easier to quit than they expected. These stages are influenced by increased costs from tax increases or reduction of smuggling, illness in the smoker, family or friends dying from tobacco, the media, health profession, bans on promotion, creation of smoke-free areas and, while most smokers still quit on their own, availability of support and treatment.

There are now techniques to assist those who want to quit smoking, although these are not available in all parts of the world: social support, clinics, quitlines, internet sites; skills training; nicotine replacement therapy (NRT) and other pharmaceutical treatments.

If interventions only focus on prevention of initiation, and do not address cessation, then 160 million additional smokers will die before 2050 (see below).

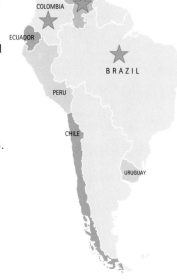

In the UK, NRT is available to all citizens under the National Health Service and is reimbursed as any other medicine.

Quitting Calendar
The benefits of stopping smoking

1 day later	Heart, blood pressure, and the blood show improvements
1 year later	Excess risk of coronary heart disease is half that of a continuing smoker
5 to 15 years later	Risk of a stroke is reduced to that of never-smokers
10 years later	Risk of lung cancer is reduced to less than half that of continuing smokers; risks of many other cancers decrease
15 years later	Risk of coronary heart disease is similar to that of never-smokers, and the overall risk of death almost the same, especially if the smoker quits before illness develops

Effects of starting and quitting smoking on deaths
Total accumulated tobacco deaths
2000, 2025 and 2050 projected
millions

if present smoking patterns continue...
70m 220m 520m

if youth uptake halves...
70m 220m 500m

if adult consumption halves...
70m 150m 340m

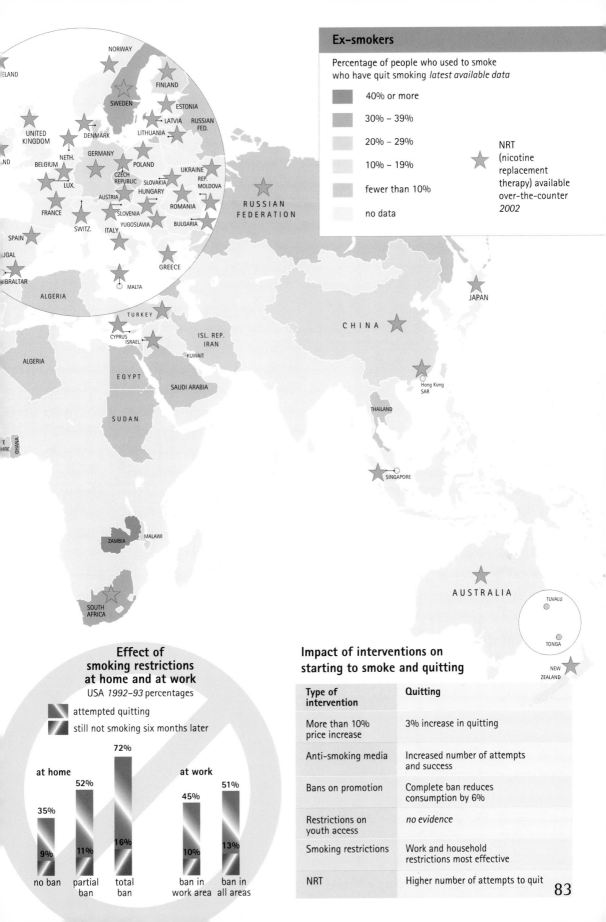

Ex-smokers

Percentage of people who used to smoke
who have quit smoking *latest available data*

- 40% or more
- 30% – 39%
- 20% – 29%
- 10% – 19%
- fewer than 10%
- no data

NRT
(nicotine
replacement
therapy) available
over-the-counter
2002

Map labels:

ELAND, NORWAY, FINLAND, SWEDEN, ESTONIA, LATVIA, RUSSIAN FED., LITHUANIA, UNITED KINGDOM, DENMARK, NETH., GERMANY, POLAND, UKRAINE, REP. MOLDOVA, BELGIUM, LUX., CZECH REPUBLIC, SLOVAKIA, HUNGARY, AUSTRIA, SLOVENIA, ROMANIA, FRANCE, SWITZ., ITALY, YUGOSLAVIA, BULGARIA, SPAIN, GREECE, JGAL, GIBRALTAR, MALTA, ALGERIA, TURKEY, CYPRUS, ISRAEL, ISL. REP. IRAN, KUWAIT, RUSSIAN FEDERATION, JAPAN, CHINA, Hong Kong SAR, THAILAND, ALGERIA, EGYPT, SAUDI ARABIA, SUDAN, E HIRE, GHANA, SINGAPORE, ZAMBIA, MALAWI, SOUTH AFRICA, AUSTRALIA, TUVALU, TONGA, NEW ZEALAND

Effect of smoking restrictions at home and at work

USA *1992–93* percentages

- attempted quitting
- still not smoking six months later

at home

- no ban: 35% / 9%
- partial ban: 52% / 11%
- total ban: 72% / 16%

at work

- ban in work area: 45% / 10%
- ban in all areas: 51% / 13%

Impact of interventions on starting to smoke and quitting

Type of intervention	Quitting
More than 10% price increase	3% increase in quitting
Anti-smoking media	Increased number of attempts and success
Bans on promotion	Complete ban reduces consumption by 6%
Restrictions on youth access	*no evidence*
Smoking restrictions	Work and household restrictions most effective
NRT	Higher number of attempts to quit

Price Policy

> "Sugar, rum and tobacco are commodities which are nowhere necessaries of life, which are become objects of almost universal consumption, and which are therefore extremely proper subjects of taxation."
> **Adam Smith** *An Inquiry into the Nature and Causes of the Wealth of Nations* 1776

The price of tobacco is the single largest factor influencing short term consumption patterns. More importantly, price plays a major role in determining how many young people will start smoking, and thus profoundly influences longterm consumption trends.

There is a clear inverse relationship between tobacco taxes and tobacco consumption. For every 10 percent increase in cigarette taxes, there is on average a four percent reduction in consumption. Youth, minorities, and low-income smokers are two to three times more likely to quit or smoke less than other smokers in response to price increases.

Tobacco taxes are an important source of revenue for countries, but the percentage of total government revenues accounted for by tobacco taxes is relatively small, less than 10 percent in all countries, and less than 2 percent in most countries. Higher tobacco taxes are also easy to implement, and nearly always provide more government revenue, despite the fact that people are smoking less.

CANADA $2

UNITED STATES OF AMERICA various states

MEXICO
JAMAICA
EL SALVADOR
COSTA RICA
VENEZUELA
COLOMBIA
ECUADOR
PERU
BRAZIL
BOLIVIA
CHILE
URUGUAY
ARGENTINA

Tax down – but prices up
Declining cigarette tax in the USA as a percentage of retail price
Smokers often assume that cigarettes have become so expensive because of increased taxes. In fact, in the USA, while the price of cigarettes has increased, the proportion going to tax is half of what it was in 1965.

1965	1970	1975	1980	1985	1990	1995	2000
51%	47%	41%	33%	31%	26%	32%	24%

Smoking goes down as prices go up
Real cigarette prices and cigarette consumption in the UK *1971–95*

expenditure on cigarettes in millions of pounds sterling

price of 20 cigarettes

	1971	1974	1977	1980	1983	1986	1989	1992	1995
expenditure	14,600	16,200	13,900	14,900	12,400	11,500	11,300	10,500	9,900
price	£1.75	£1.50	£1.80	£1.55	£1.84	£2.14	£2.01	£2.20	£2.60

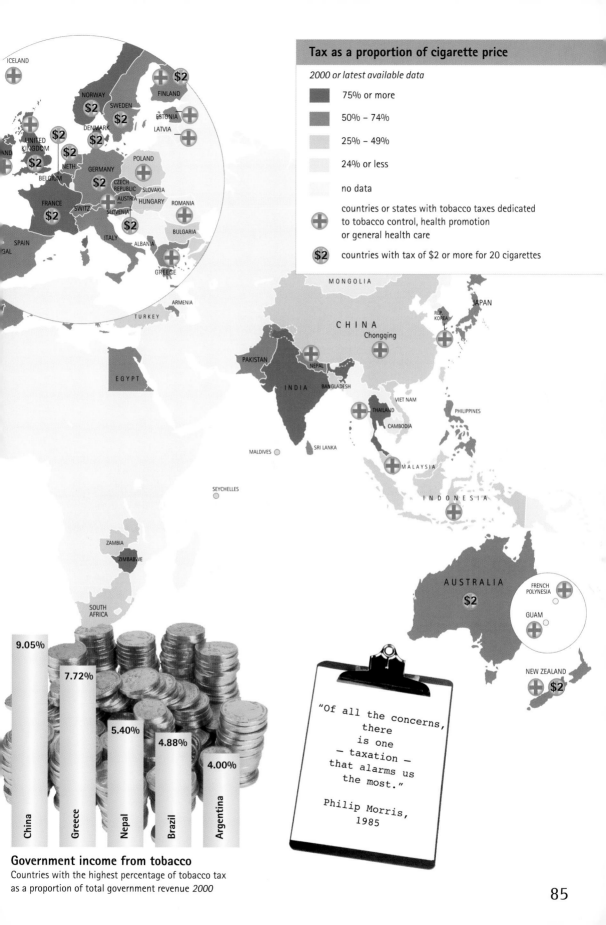

Tax as a proportion of cigarette price

2000 or latest available data

- 75% or more
- 50% – 74%
- 25% – 49%
- 24% or less
- no data
- ⊕ countries or states with tobacco taxes dedicated to tobacco control, health promotion or general health care
- $2 countries with tax of $2 or more for 20 cigarettes

ICELAND

NORWAY $2
SWEDEN $2
FINLAND $2
DENMARK $2
ESTONIA
LATVIA
UNITED KINGDOM $2
$2
NETH. $2
BELGIUM
GERMANY $2
POLAND
CZECH REPUBLIC
SLOVAKIA
FRANCE $2
SWITZ.
AUSTRIA
SLOVENIA
HUNGARY
ROMANIA
ITALY $2
SPAIN
ALBANIA
BULGARIA
GREECE
GAL
ARMENIA
TURKEY
EGYPT

MONGOLIA
JAPAN
REP. KOREA
CHINA
Chongqing
PAKISTAN ⊕
NEPAL
INDIA
BANGLADESH
VIET NAM
THAILAND ⊕
CAMBODIA
PHILIPPINES
SRI LANKA
MALDIVES ○
MALAYSIA ⊕
SEYCHELLES ○
INDONESIA ⊕

ZAMBIA
ZIMBABWE
SOUTH AFRICA

AUSTRALIA $2

FRENCH POLYNESIA ⊕
GUAM ⊕

NEW ZEALAND ⊕ $2

"Of all the concerns, there is one — taxation — that alarms us the most."

Philip Morris, 1985

Government income from tobacco

China 9.05%
Greece 7.72%
Nepal 5.40%
Brazil 4.88%
Argentina 4.00%

Countries with the highest percentage of tobacco tax as a proportion of total government revenue *2000*

Litigation

Tobacco litigation began with a personal injury lawsuit in the USA in 1954. For more than 40 years, the tobacco industry boasted it had not lost a single case, but this has changed. One case in Minnesota that began in 1994 ruled that millions of pages of internal tobacco industry documents (see map 21) be put into the public domain. These showed that the industry has concealed information on the true harmfulness of smoking and misled governments, the media and their clients – smokers.

Litigation has put the industry on the political defensive, forced tobacco companies to the bargaining table, and has resulted in some large settlements, with the industry paying US states billions of dollars a year.

Outside the USA, tobacco litigation is a new phenomenon, and clear patterns do not yet exist. However, some recent cases show the potential for litigation to advance tobacco control. Australia has seen a major ruling on the dangers of passive smoking. Public interest writ litigation in India has prompted the Supreme Court of India to require nationwide implementation of broad restrictions on public smoking.

Cases now vary from smokers and non-smokers filing for damage to health; public interest law suits seeking to force the industry or government to comply with legal or constitutional requirements; governments suing for tobacco-attributable health care costs or for lost taxation due to smuggling; to cases brought by the tobacco industry against individuals, organisations or even governments.

The judge in an Australian lawsuit against BAT in 2002 found "that given the fact that not a single document was in fact discovered in that category (pharmacological effects of nicotine) the implication seems overwhelming that discovery has been fundamentally thwarted under this category by virtue of the 1998 destruction programme."

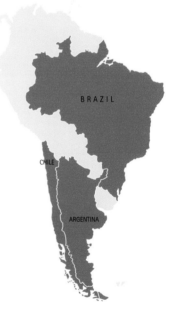

BAT faced

4,419

lawsuits
in the USA alone
at the end of 2001

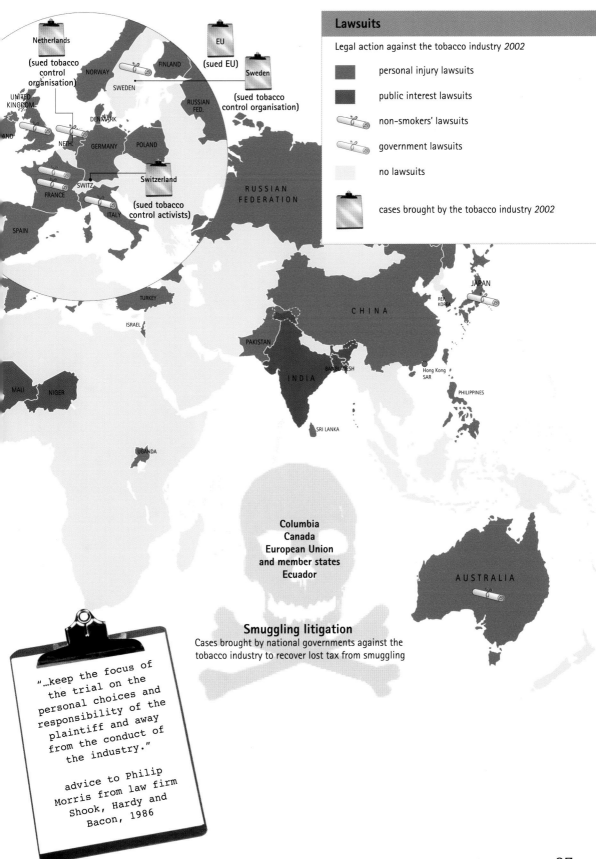

Lawsuits

Legal action against the tobacco industry *2002*

- personal injury lawsuits
- public interest lawsuits
- non-smokers' lawsuits
- government lawsuits
- no lawsuits
- cases brought by the tobacco industry *2002*

Netherlands
(sued tobacco control organisation)

EU
(sued EU)

Sweden
(sued tobacco control organisation)

Switzerland
(sued tobacco control activists)

Smuggling litigation
Cases brought by national governments against the tobacco industry to recover lost tax from smuggling

Columbia
Canada
European Union
and member states
Ecuador

"...keep the focus of the trial on the personal choices and responsibility of the plaintiff and away from the conduct of the industry."

advice to Philip Morris from law firm Shook, Hardy and Bacon, 1986

Projections by Industry

The tobacco industry predicts a global expansion of the tobacco epidemic in the next few years. The increases in consumption lie principally in the developing nations, while consumption in the industrialised countries will be static or in decline.

In all the countries surveyed, the biggest growth between 1998 and 2008 is expected to be in Zimbabwe, followed by Côte d'Ivoire, Brazil, Morocco, Venezuela, Pakistan, United Republic of Tanzania and Bangladesh.

The greatest decline is expected in New Zealand, followed by the UK, South Africa, Hong Kong, Australia, Singapore and Finland.

In Africa, only the South African market is expected to decrease.

In the Americas, growth in Latin America is expected to compensate for declines in the USA and Canada, with the greatest increases in Brazil, Venezuela, Mexico, Peru, Chile and Uruguay.

In Europe, the forecast is mixed, with increases in some markets and decreases in others. The biggest increase is expected in Norway, and the greatest decline in the UK.

In the Middle East region, the highest growth is expected for Morocco, followed by Pakistan and Tunisia. No country in this region is expected to experience a decline in consumption.

In South East Asia, Bangladesh will see the highest growth, followed by Thailand, while consumption remains static in India.

In the Western Pacific, Vietnam tops the growth charts, while New Zealand, Hong Kong, Australia and Singapore show the greatest decline.

This transfer of the epidemic from rich to poor countries, with its health and economic consequences, is one that developing countries can ill afford. As long ago as 1986, the World Health Organization predicted that the differential in wealth between rich and poor countries would widen further as a result of tobacco, leading to compromise in sustainable development.

These projections are not inevitable; tobacco control interventions can make a difference.

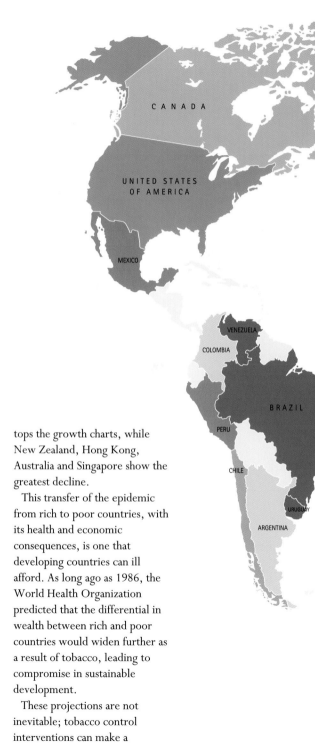

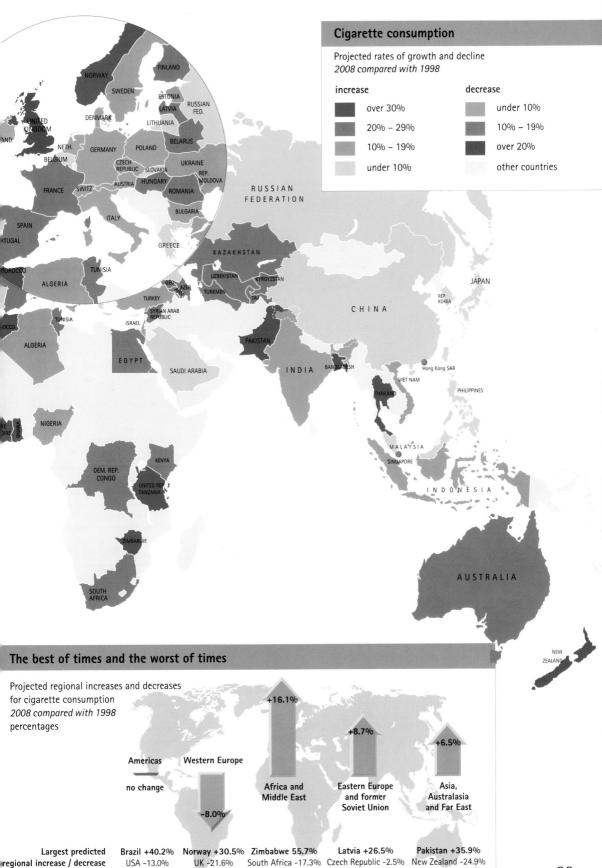

Cigarette consumption

Projected rates of growth and decline
2008 compared with 1998

increase
- over 30%
- 20% – 29%
- 10% – 19%
- under 10%

decrease
- under 10%
- 10% – 19%
- over 20%
- other countries

The best of times and the worst of times

Projected regional increases and decreases
for cigarette consumption
2008 compared with 1998
percentages

Americas — no change

Western Europe **−8.0%**

Africa and Middle East **+16.1%**

Eastern Europe and former Soviet Union **+8.7%**

Asia, Australasia and Far East **+6.5%**

Largest predicted regional increase / decrease

	Americas	Western Europe	Africa and Middle East	Eastern Europe and former Soviet Union	Asia, Australasia and Far East
increase	Brazil +40.2%	Norway +30.5%	Zimbabwe 55.7%	Latvia +26.5%	Pakistan +35.9%
decrease	USA -13.0%	UK -21.6%	South Africa -17.3%	Czech Republic -2.5%	New Zealand -24.9%

89

The Future

Future predictions are by their nature speculative but some things are certain: the tobacco epidemic, with its attendant health and economic burden, is both increasing and also shifting from developed to developing nations nations; and more women are smoking.

The industry is consolidating, and also shifting from the west to developing regions, where there may be less government control and public debate about the role of transnational tobacco companies.

The future looks bleak; the global tobacco epidemic is worse today than it was 50 years ago. And it will be even worse in another 50 years unless an extraordinary effort is made now. Several countries have already shown that smoking rates can be reduced. These successes can be reproduced by any responsible nation, but only through immediate, determined, and sustained governmental and community action. The future epidemic depends on understanding of the issue, and policies, politics and actions taken today.

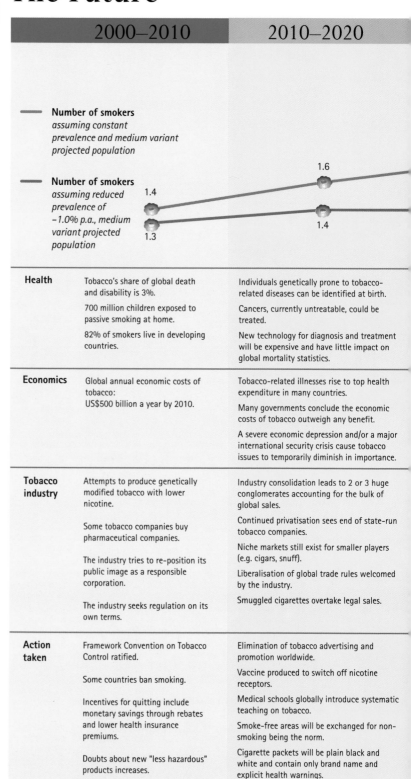

	2000–2010	2010–2020
Health	Tobacco's share of global death and disability is 3%. 700 million children exposed to passive smoking at home. 82% of smokers live in developing countries.	Individuals genetically prone to tobacco-related diseases can be identified at birth. Cancers, currently untreatable, could be treated. New technology for diagnosis and treatment will be expensive and have little impact on global mortality statistics.
Economics	Global annual economic costs of tobacco: US$500 billion a year by 2010.	Tobacco-related illnesses rise to top health expenditure in many countries. Many governments conclude the economic costs of tobacco outweigh any benefit. A severe economic depression and/or a major international security crisis cause tobacco issues to temporarily diminish in importance.
Tobacco industry	Attempts to produce genetically modified tobacco with lower nicotine. Some tobacco companies buy pharmaceutical companies. The industry tries to re-position its public image as a responsible corporation. The industry seeks regulation on its own terms.	Industry consolidation leads to 2 or 3 huge conglomerates accounting for the bulk of global sales. Continued privatisation sees end of state-run tobacco companies. Niche markets still exist for smaller players (e.g. cigars, snuff). Liberalisation of global trade rules welcomed by the industry. Smuggled cigarettes overtake legal sales.
Action taken	Framework Convention on Tobacco Control ratified. Some countries ban smoking. Incentives for quitting include monetary savings through rebates and lower health insurance premiums. Doubts about new "less hazardous" products increases. In developed countries, there is a gradual shift in the perception of smoking as it comes to be seen as anti-social.	Elimination of tobacco advertising and promotion worldwide. Vaccine produced to switch off nicotine receptors. Medical schools globally introduce systematic teaching on tobacco. Smoke-free areas will be exchanged for non-smoking being the norm. Cigarette packets will be plain black and white and contain only brand name and explicit health warnings. Tobacco dependent economies are assisted in diversifying. Nicotine Replacement Therapy sold over the counter worldwide.

Within the chart area:

Number of smokers *assuming constant prevalence and medium variant projected population*

Number of smokers *assuming reduced prevalence of –1.0% p.a., medium variant projected population*

1.4

1.3

1.6

1.4

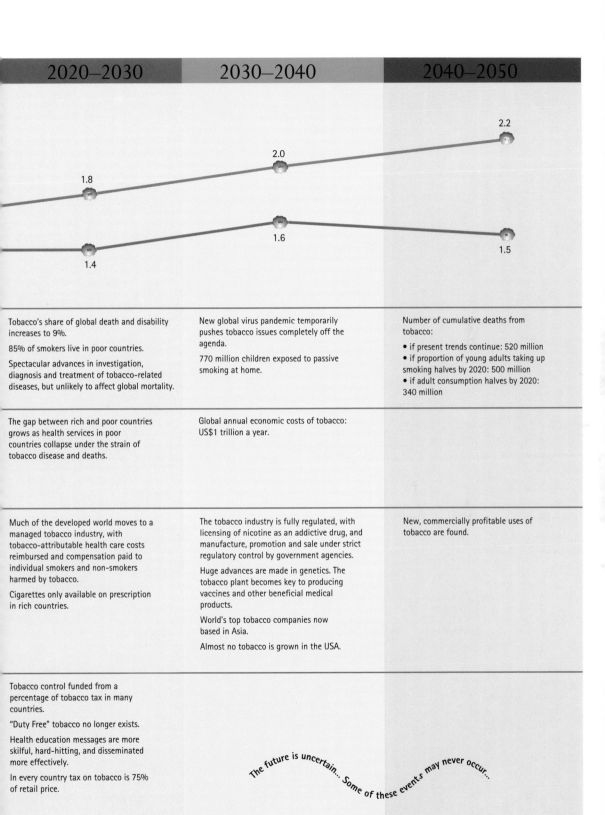

| 2020–2030 | 2030–2040 | 2040–2050 |

1.8

2.0

2.2

1.4

1.6

1.5

Tobacco's share of global death and disability increases to 9%.

85% of smokers live in poor countries.

Spectacular advances in investigation, diagnosis and treatment of tobacco-related diseases, but unlikely to affect global mortality.

New global virus pandemic temporarily pushes tobacco issues completely off the agenda.

770 million children exposed to passive smoking at home.

Number of cumulative deaths from tobacco:

• if present trends continue: 520 million
• if proportion of young adults taking up smoking halves by 2020: 500 million
• if adult consumption halves by 2020: 340 million

The gap between rich and poor countries grows as health services in poor countries collapse under the strain of tobacco disease and deaths.

Global annual economic costs of tobacco: US$1 trillion a year.

Much of the developed world moves to a managed tobacco industry, with tobacco-attributable health care costs reimbursed and compensation paid to individual smokers and non-smokers harmed by tobacco.

Cigarettes only available on prescription in rich countries.

The tobacco industry is fully regulated, with licensing of nicotine as an addictive drug, and manufacture, promotion and sale under strict regulatory control by government agencies.

Huge advances are made in genetics. The tobacco plant becomes key to producing vaccines and other beneficial medical products.

World's top tobacco companies now based in Asia.

Almost no tobacco is grown in the USA.

New, commercially profitable uses of tobacco are found.

Tobacco control funded from a percentage of tobacco tax in many countries.

"Duty Free" tobacco no longer exists.

Health education messages are more skilful, hard-hitting, and disseminated more effectively.

In every country tax on tobacco is 75% of retail price.

The future is uncertain... Some of these events may never occur...

91

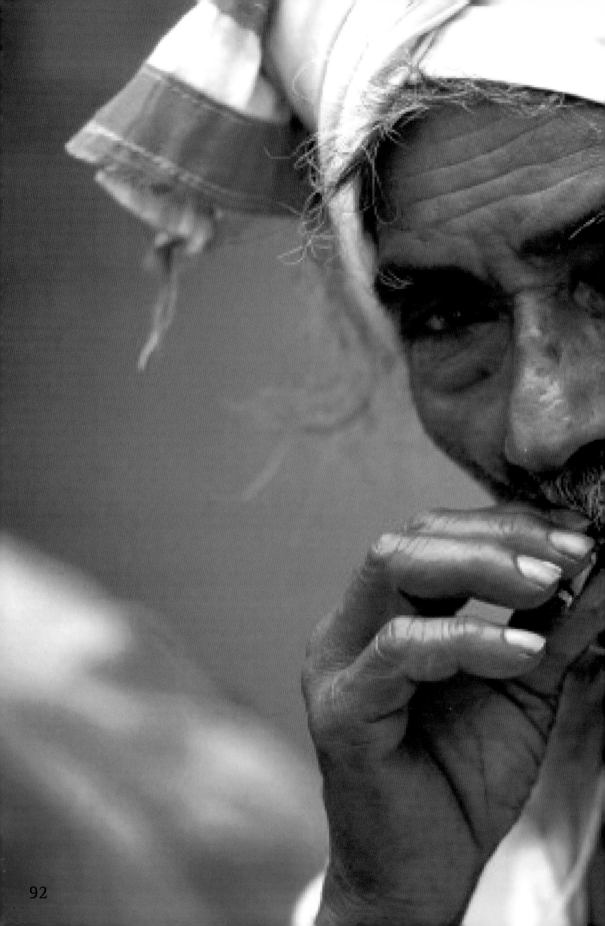

PART 6

WORLD TABLES

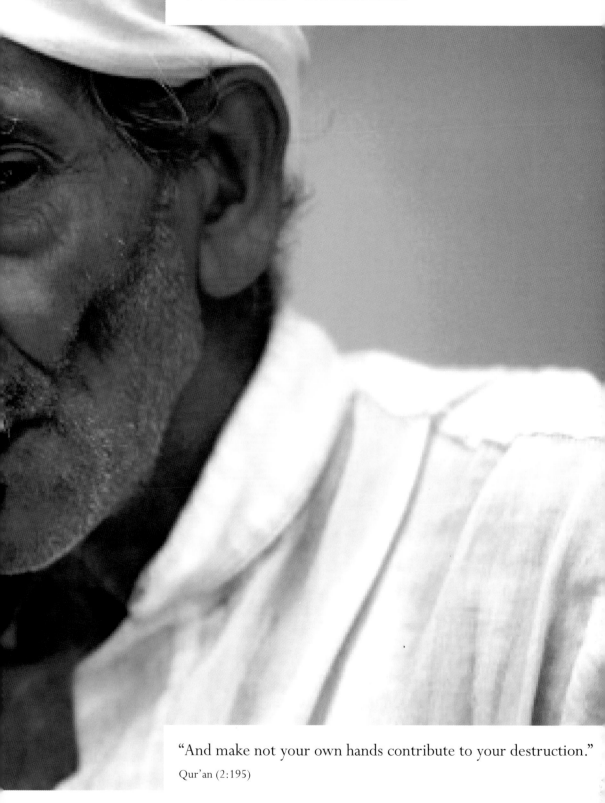

"And make not your own hands contribute to your destruction."
Qur'an (2:195)

The Demographics of Tobacco

Countries	1 Population	2 Adult smoking			3 Youth tobacco use [1]		
	thousands	total	percentages male	female	total	percentages male	female
Afghanistan	21,765	–	–	–	–	–	–
Albania	3,134	39.0%	60.0%	18.0%	–	–	–
Algeria	30,291	25.2%	43.8%	6.6%	–	–	–
Andorra	86	35.9%	43.7%	28%	–	–	–
Angola	13,134	–	–	–	–	–	–
Antigua and Barbuda	65	–	–	–	13.0%	13.8%	11.8%
Argentina	37,032	40.4%	46.8%	34.0%	28.1%	25.7%	30.0%
Armenia	3,787	32.5%	64.0%	1.0%	–	–	–
Australia	19,138	19.5%	21.1%	18.0%	–	–	–
Austria	8,080	24.5%	30.0%	19.0%	–	–	–
Azerbaijan	8,041	15.7%	30.2%	1.1%	–	–	–
Bahamas	304	11.5%	19.0%	4.0%	16.0%	20.0%	12.6%
Bahrain	640	14.6%	23.5%	5.7%	–	–	–
Bangladesh	137,439	38.7%	53.6%	23.8%	–	–	–
Barbados	267	9.0%	–	–	16.9%	15.9%	17.7%
Belarus	10,187	29.8%	54.9%	4.6%	–	–	–
Belgium	10,249	28.0%	30.0%	26.0%	–	–	–
Belize	226	–	–	–	–	–	–
Benin	6,272	37.0%	–	–	–	–	–
Bhutan	2,085	–	–	–	–	–	–
Bolivia	8,329	30.4%	42.7%	18.1%	26.4%	31.0%	22.0%
Bosnia and Herzegovina	3,977	48.0%	–	–	–	–	–
Botswana	1,541	21.0%	–	–	–	–	–
Brazil	170,406	33.8%	38.2%	29.3%	–	–	–
Brunei Darussalam	328	27.0%	40.0%	14.0%	–	–	–
Bulgaria	7,949	36.5%	49.2%	23.8%	–	–	–
Burkina Faso	11,535	–	–	–	–	–	–
Burundi	6,356	–	–	–	–	–	–
Cambodia	13,104	37.0%	66.0%	8.0%	–	–	–
Cameroon	14,876	35.7%	–	–	–	–	–
Canada	30,757	25.0%	27.0%	23.0%	–	–	–
Cape Verde	427	–	–	–	–	–	–
Central African Rep.	3,717	–	–	–	–	–	–
Chad	7,885	–	24.1%	–	–	–	–
Chile	15,211	22.2%	26.0%	18.3%	37.9%	34.0%	43.4%
China	1,282,437	35.6%	66.9%	4.2%	10.8%	14.0%	7.0%
Colombia	42,105	22.3%	23.5%	21.0%	–	–	–
Comoros	706	–	–	–	–	–	–
Congo	3,018	–	–	–	–	–	–
Congo, Dem. Rep.	50,948	–	–	5.5%	–	–	–
Cook Islands	20	28.5%	40.0%	17.0%	–	–	–
Costa Rica	4,024	17.6%	28.6%	6.6%	20.8%	20.6%	21.0%
Côte d'Ivoire	16,013	22.1%	42.3%	1.8%	–	–	–
Croatia	4,654	33.0%	34.0%	32.0%	–	–	–
Cuba	11,199	37.2%	48.0%	26.3%	19.2%	18.0%	20.0%
Cyprus	784	23.1%	38.5%	7.6%	–	–	–
Czech Republic	10,272	29%	36.0%	22.0%	–	–	–
Denmark	5,320	30.5%	32.0%	29.0%	–	–	–

Sources: see page 124

[1] For some countries, data are based on youth surveys in major cities or province and are not necessarily representative of the entire countr

4 Youth exposed to passive smoking at home [2] percentages	5 Cigarette consumption annual per person	6 Quitting percentages of people who quit smoking by 2002	Countries
–	98	–	Afghanistan
–	–	–	Albania
–	1,021	29%	Algeria
–	–	–	Andorra
–	571	–	Angola
17.4%	–	–	Antigua and Barbuda
68.2%	1,495	–	Argentina
–	1,095	–	Armenia
–	1,907	–	Australia
–	2,073	18%	Austria
–	1,150	–	Azerbaijan
28.7%	613	15%	Bahamas
–	2,179	–	Bahrain
–	245	–	Bangladesh
22.9%	542	–	Barbados
–	2,571	–	Belarus
–	2,428	–	Belgium
–	1,092	–	Belize
–	–	–	Benin
–	–	–	Bhutan
46.0%	274	–	Bolivia
–	–	–	Bosnia and Herzegovina
–	–	–	Botswana
–	858	–	Brazil
–	–	–	Brunei Darussalam
–	2,574	–	Bulgaria
–	221	–	Burkina Faso
–	86	–	Burundi
–	–	–	Cambodia
–	652	–	Cameroon
–	1,976	–	Canada
–	–	–	Cape Verde
–	329	–	Central African Rep.
–	160	–	Chad
57.0%	1,202	35%	Chile
53.0%	1,791	10%	China
–	521	–	Colombia
–	–	–	Comoros
–	476	–	Congo
–	135	–	Congo, Dem. Rep.
–	–	–	Cook Islands
32.8%	690	–	Costa Rica
–	580	11%	Côte d'Ivoire
–	1,995	–	Croatia
68.9%	1,343	–	Cuba
–	–	11%	Cyprus
–	2,306	24%	Czech Republic
–	1,919	20%	Denmark

For some countries, data are based on youth surveys in major cities or provinces, and are not necessarily representative of the entire country.

95

Countries	1 Population	2 Adult smoking			3 Youth tobacco use [1]		
	thousands	total	percentages male	female	total	percentages male	female
Djibouti	632	31.1%	57.5%	4.7%	–	–	–
Dominica	71	–	–	–	19.3%	23.8%	14.5%
Dominican Republic	8,373	20.7%	24.3%	17.1%	–	–	–
East Timor		––	–	–	–	–	–
Ecuador	12,646	31.5%	45.5%	17.4%	–	–	–
Egypt	67,884	18.3%	35.0%	1.6%	–	–	–
El Salvador	6,278	25.0%	38.0%	12.0%	–	–	–
Equatorial Guinea	457	–	–	–	–	–	–
Eritrea	3,659	–	–	–	–	–	–
Estonia	1,393	32.0%	44.0%	20.0%	–	–	–
Ethiopia	62,908	15.8%	–	–	–	–	–
Fiji	814	20.5%	24.0%	17.0%	15.1%	19.3%	10.9%
Finland	5,172	23.5%	27.0%	20.0%	–	–	–
France	59,238	34.5%	38.6%	30.3%	–	–	–
Gabon	1,230	–	–	–	–	–	–
Gambia	1,303	17.8%	34.0%	1.5%	–	–	–
Georgia	5,262	37.5%	60.0%	15.0%	–	–	–
Germany	82,017	35.0%	39.0%	31.0%	–	–	–
Ghana	19,306	16.0%	28.4%	3.5%	16.8%	16.2%	17.3%
Greece	10,610	38.0%	47.0%	29.0%	–	–	–
Grenada	94	–	–	–	14.4%	17.0%	11.9%
Guatemala	11,385	27.8%	37.8%	17.7%	–	–	–
Guinea	8,154	51.7%	59.5%	43.8%	–	–	–
Guinea-Bissau	1,199–	–	–	–	–	–	–
Guyana	761	–	–	–	15.3%	21.6%	11.1%
Haiti	8,142	9.7%	10.7%	8.6%	20.7%	21.0%	20.0%
Honduras	6,417	23.5%	36.0%	11.0%	–	–	–
Hungary	9,968	35.5%	44.0%	27.0%	–	–	–
Iceland	279	24.0%	25.0%	23.0%	–	–	–
India	1,008,937	16.0%	29.4%	2.5%	variable	variable	variable
Indonesia	212,092	31.4%	59.0%	3.7%	22.0%	38.0%	5.3%
Iran, Isl. Rep.	70,330	15.3%	27.2%	3.4%	–	–	–
Iraq	22,946	22.5%	40.0%	5.0%	–	–	–
Ireland	3,803	31.5%	32.0%	31.0%	–	–	–
Israel	6,040	28.5%	33.0%	24.0%	–	–	–
Italy	57,530	24.9%	32.4%	17.3%	–	–	–
Jamaica	2,576	14.6%	–	–	19.3%	24.4%	14.5%
Japan	127,096	33.1%	52.8%	13.4%	–	–	–
Jordan	4,913	29.0%	48.0%	10.0%	20.6%	27.0%	13.4%
Kazakhstan	16,172	33.5%	60.0%	7.0%	–	–	–
Kenya	30,669	49.4%	66.8%	31.9%	13.0%	16.0%	10.0%
Kiribati	83	42.0%	56.5%	32.3%	–	–	–
Korea, Republic of	46,740	35.0%	65.1%	4.8%	–	–	–
Korea, Dem. People's Rep. of	22,268	–	–	–	–	–	–
Kuwait	1,914	15.6%	29.6%	1.5%	–	–	–
Kyrgyzstan	4,921	37.8%	60.0%	15.6%	–	–	–
Lao People's Dem. Rep.	5,279	38.0%	41.0%	15.0%	–	–	–
Latvia	2,421	31.0%	49.0%	13.0%	–	–	–

Sources: see page 124

[1] For some countries, data are based on youth surveys in major cities or provin
and are not necessarily representative of the entire cour

4 Youth exposed to passive smoking at home [2] percentages	5 Cigarette consumption annual per person	6 Quitting percentages of people who quit smoking by 2002	Countries
–	–	–	Djibouti
27.4%	–	–	Dominica
–	754	11%	Dominican Republic
–	–	–	East Timor
–	232	31%	Ecuador
–	1,275	5%	Egypt
–	429	–	El Salvador
–	–	–	Equatorial Guinea
–	–	–	Eritrea
–	1,983	–	Estonia
–	87	–	Ethiopia
49.4%	976	–	Fiji
–	1,351	16%	Finland
–	2,058	–	France
–	487	–	Gabon
–	171	–	Gambia
–	–	–	Georgia
–	1,702	18%	Germany
22.2%	161	3%	Ghana
–	4,313	–	Greece
28.9%	–	–	Grenada
–	609	–	Guatemala
–	–	–	Guinea
–	90	–	Guinea-Bissau
31.6%	590	–	Guyana
31.3%	172	–	Haiti
–	595	40%	Honduras
–	3,265	–	Hungary
–	1,915	–	Iceland
34.3%	129	–	India
63.0%	1,742	–	Indonesia
–	765	20%	Iran, Isl. Rep.
–	1,430	–	Iraq
–	2,236	–	Ireland
–	2,162	10%	Israel
–	1,901	–	Italy
30.8%	735	–	Jamaica
–	3,023	–	Japan
67.4%	1,832	–	Jordan
–	2,160	–	Kazakhstan
29.5%	200	–	Kenya
–	–	–	Kiribati
–	2,918	–	Korea, Republic of
–	–	–	Korea, Dem. People's Rep. of
–	3,062	9%	Kuwait
–	1,886	–	Kyrgyzstan
–	400	–	Lao People's Dem. Rep.
–	–	–	Latvia

For some countries, data are based on youth surveys in major cities or provinces,
and are not necessarily representative of the entire country.

The Demographics of Tobacco

Countries	1 Population thousands	2 Adult smoking			3 Youth tobacco use [1]		
		total	percentages male	female	total	percentages male	female
Lebanon	3,496	40.5%	46.0%	35.0%	–	–	–
Lesotho	2,035	19.8%	38.5%	1.0%	–	–	–
Liberia	2,913	–	–	–	–	–	–
Libyan Arab Jamahiriya	5,290	4.0%	–	–	–	–	–
Lithuania	3,696	33.5%	51.0%	16.0%	–	–	–
Luxembourg	437	33.0%	39.0%	27.0%	–	–	–
Macedonia, Former Yugos. Rep. of	2,034	36.0%	40.0%	32.0%	–	–	–
Madagascar	15,970	–	–	–	–	–	–
Malawi	11,308	14.5%	20.0%	9.0%	16.8%	18.0%	15.0%
Malaysia	22,218	26.4%	49.2%	3.5%	–	–	–
Maldives	291	26.0%	37.0%	15.0%	–	–	–
Mali	11,351	–	–	–	–	–	–
Malta	390	23.9%	33.1%	14.6%	–	–	–
Marshall Islands	51–	–	–	–	–	–	–
Mauritania	2,665	–	–	–	–	–	–
Mauritius	1,161	23.9%	44.8%	2.9%	–	–	–
Mexico	98,872	34.8%	51.2%	18.4%	21.7%	27.9%	16.0%
Micronesia, Federated States of	123	–	–	–	–	–	–
Moldova, Republic of	4,295	32.0%	46.0%	18.0%	–	–	–
Monaco	33	–	–	–	–	–	–
Mongolia	2,533	46.7%	67.8%	25.5%	–	–	–
Morocco	29,878	18.1%	34.5%	1.6%	–	–	–
Mozambique	18,292	–	–	–	–	–	–
Myanmar	47,749	32.9%	43.5%	22.3%	–	–	–
Namibia	1,757	50.0%	65.0%	35.0%	–	–	–
Nauru	12	54.0%	61.0%	47.0%	–	–	–
Nepal	23,043	38.5%	48.0%	29.0%	7.8%	12.0%	6.0%
Netherlands	15,864	33.0%	37.0%	29.0%	–	–	–
New Zealand	3,778	25.0%	25.0%	25.0%	–	–	–
Nicaragua	5,071	–	–	–	–	–	–
Niger	10,832	–	–	–	–	–	–
Nigeria	113,862	8.6%	15.4%	1.7%	18.1%	22.0%	16.0%
Niue	2	37.5%	58.0%	17.0%	–	–	–
Norway	4,469	31.5%	31.0%	32.0%	–	–	–
Oman	2,538	8.5%	15.5%	1.5%	–	–	–
Pakistan	141,256	22.5%	36.0%	9.0%	–	–	–
Palau	19	15.1%	22.3%	7.9%	58.5%	55.0%	62.0%
Panama	2,856	38.0%	56.0%	20.0%	–	–	–
Papua New Guinea	4,809	37.0%	46.0%	28.0%	–	–	–
Paraguay	5,496	14.8%	24.1%	5.5%	–	–	–
Peru	25,662	28.6%	41.5%	15.7%	19.5%	22.0%	15.0%
Philippines	75653	32.4%	53.8%	11.0%	23.3%	31.2%	17.2%
Poland	38,605	34.5%	44.0%	25.0%	24.4%	29.0%	20.0%
Portugal	10,016	18.7%	30.2%	7.1%	–	–	–
Qatar	565	18.8%	37.0%	0.5%	–	–	–
Romania	22,438	43.5%	62.0%	25.0%	–	–	–
Russian Federation	145,491	36.5%	63.2%	9.7%	35.1%	40.9%	29.5%
Rwanda	7,609	5.5%	7.0%	4.0%	–	–	–

 Sources: see page 124

[1] For some countries, data are based on youth surveys in major cities or provinces and are not necessarily representative of the entire country.

4 Youth exposed to passive smoking at home [2] percentages	5 Cigarette consumption annual per person	6 Quitting percentages of people who quit smoking by 2002	Countries
-	-	-	Lebanon
-	-	-	Lesotho
-	89	-	Liberia
-	1,482	-	Libyan Arab Jamahiriya
-	-	-	Lithuania
-	-	-	Luxembourg
-	-	-	Macedonia, Former Yugos. Rep. of
-	315	-	Madagascar
-	123	11%	Malawi
-	910	-	Malaysia
-	1,441	-	Maldives
60.5%	223	-	Mali
-	2,668	-	Malta
-	-	-	Marshall Islands
-	317	-	Mauritania
-	1,284	-	Mauritius
45.5%	754	15%	Mexico
-	-	-	Micronesia, Federated States of
-	2,640	-	Moldova, Republic of
-	-	-	Monaco
-	-	-	Mongolia
-	800	-	Morocco
-	432	-	Mozambique
-	-	-	Myanmar
-	-	-	Namibia
-	-	-	Nauru
37.8%	619	-	Nepal
-	2,323	-	Netherlands
-	1,213	-	New Zealand
-	793	-	Nicaragua
-	-	-	Niger
34.3%	189	-	Nigeria
-	-	-	Niue
-	725	-	Norway
-	-	-	Oman
-	564	-	Pakistan
46.0%	-	-	Palau
-	244	-	Panama
-	-	-	Papua New Guinea
-	1,748	-	Paraguay
29.0%	195	12%	Peru
58.2%	1,849	-	Philippines
67.0%	2,061	-	Poland
-	2,079	-	Portugal
-	-	-	Qatar
-	1,676	-	Romania
55.3%	1,702	1%	Russian Federation
-	135	-	Rwanda

For some countries, data are based on youth surveys in major cities or provinces,
and are not necessarily representative of the entire country.

The Demographics of Tobacco

Countries	1 Population	2 Adult smoking			3 Youth tobacco use [1]		
	thousands	total	percentages male	female	total	percentages male	female
Saint Kitts and Nevis	38	–	–	–	–	–	–
Saint Lucia	148	–	–	–	–	–	–
Saint Vincent and Grenadines	113	15%	26.4%	3.5%	–	–	–
Samoa	159	23.3%	33.9%	12.7%	–	–	–
San Marino	27	22.5%	28.0%	17.0%	–	–	–
Sao Tome and Principe	138	44.1%	–	–	–	–	–
Saudi Arabia	20,346	11.5%	22.0%	1.0%	–	–	–
Senegal	9,421	4.6%	–	–	–	–	–
Seychelles	80	22.0%	37.0%	6.9%	–	–	–
Sierra Leone	4,405	18.5%	–	–	–	–	–
Singapore	4,018	15.0%	26.9%	3.1%	9.1%	10.5%	7.5%
Slovakia	5,399	42.6%	55.1%	30.0%	–	–	–
Slovenia	1,988	25.2%	30.0%	20.3%	–	–	–
Solomon Islands	447	–	–	23.0%	–	–	–
Somalia	8,778	–	–	–	–	–	–
South Africa	43,309	26.5%	42.0%	11.0%	24.3%	29.0%	20.8%
Spain	39,910	33.4%	42.1%	24.7%	–	–	–
Sri Lanka	18,924	13.7%	25.7%	1.7%	9.9%	13.7%	5.8%
Sudan	31,095	12.9%	24.4%	1.4%	–	–	–
Suriname	417	–	–	–	14.3%	18.5%	10.1%
Swaziland	925	13.4%	24.7%	2.1%	–	–	–
Sweden	8,842	19.0%	19.0%	19.0%	–	–	–
Switzerland	7,170	33.5%	39.0%	28.0%	–	–	–
Syrian Arab Republic	16,189	30.3%	50.6%	9.9%	–	–	–
Tajikistan	6,087	–	–	–	–	–	–
Tanzania, United Republic of	35,119	31.0%	49.5%	12.4%	–	–	–
Thailand	62,806	23.4%	44.1%	2.6%	–	–	–
Togo	4,527	–	–	–	–	–	–
Tonga	99	38.3%	62.4%	14.2%	–	–	–
Trinidad and Tobago	1,294	25.1%	42.1%	8.0%	14.2%	17.9%	10.2%
Tunisia	9,459	34.8%	61.9%	7.7%	–	–	–
Turkey	66,668	44.0%	60–65%	20–24%	–	–	–
Turkmenistan	4,737	14.0%	27.0%	1.0%	–	–	–
Tuvalu	10	41.0%	51.0%	31.0%	–	–	–
Uganda	23,300	34.5%	52.0%	17.0%	–	–	–
Ukraine	49,568	35.3%	51.1%	19.4%	34.6%	37.7%	30.8%
United Arab Emirates	2,606	9.0%	18.3%	<1.0%	–	–	–
United Kingdom	59,415	26.5%	27.0%	26.0%	–	–	–
United States of America	283,230	23.6%	25.7%	21.5%	25.8%	27.5%	24.2%
Uruguay	3,337	23.0%	31.7%	14.3%	23.9%	22.0%	24.0%
Uzbekistan	24,881	29.0%	49.0%	9.0%	–	–	–
Vanuatu	197	27.0%	49.0%	5.0%	–	–	–
Venezuela	24,170	40.5%	41.8%	39.2%	14.8%	15.3%	13.9%
Viet Nam	78,137	27.1%	50.7%	3.5%	–	–	–
Yemen	18,349	44.5%	60.0%	29.0%	–	–	–
Yugoslavia	10,552	47.0%	52.0%	42.0%	–	–	–
Zambia	10,421	22.5%	35.0%	10.0%	–	–	–
Zimbabwe	12,627	17.8%	34.4%	1.2%	18.3%	19.0%	17.0%

Sources: see page 124

[1] For some countries, data are based on youth surveys in major cities or provinc
and are not necessarily representative of the entire count

4 Youth exposed to passive smoking at home [2] percentages	5 Cigarette consumption annual per person	6 Quitting percentages of people who quit smoking by 2002	Countries
-	-	-	Saint Kitts and Nevis
26.9%	-	-	Saint Lucia
32.5%	-	-	Saint Vincent and Grenadines
-	1,509	-	Samoa
-	-	-	San Marino
-	-	-	Sao Tome and Principe
-	810	9%	Saudi Arabia-
-	340	-	Senegal
-	-	-	Seychelles-
-	465	-	Sierra Leone
35.1%	1,230	-	Singapore
-	2,282	-	Slovakia
-	2,917	-	Slovenia
-	678	-	Solomon Islands
-	-	-	Somalia
43.6%	1,516	35%	South Africa
-	2,779	-	Spain
55.8%	374	-	Sri Lanka
30.5%	77	1%	Sudan
56.6%	1,930	-	Suriname
-	-	-	Swaziland
-	1,202	33%	Sweden
-	2,720	-	Switzerland
-	1,283	-	Syrian Arab Republic
-	-	-	Tajikistan
-	177	-	Tanzania, United Republic of
-	1,067	1%	Thailand
-	306	-	Togo
-	-	5%	Tonga
37.2%	2,180	13%	Trinidad and Tobago
-	1,341	-	Tunisia
-	2,394	10%	Turkey
-	2,307	-	Turkmenistan
-	-	5%	Tuvalu
-	180	-	Uganda
49.0%	1,456	-	Ukraine
-	-	-	United Arab Emirates
-	1,748	-	United Kingdom
42.1%	2,255	42%	United States of America
-	1,396	16%	Uruguay
-	1,104	-	Uzbekistan
-	-	-	Vanuatu
43.5%	1,079	7%	Venezuela
-	1,025	-	Viet Nam
-	-	-	Yemen
-	1,548	-	Yugoslavia
-	408	72%	Zambia
35.6%	399	-	Zimbabwe

For some countries, data are based on youth surveys in major cities or provinces, and are not necessarily representative of the entire country.

Table B The Business of Tobacco

Countries	1 Growing Tobacco			2 Tobacco Trade			
	Land devoted to growing tobacco hectares	Agricultural land devoted to tobacco farming percentage of total	Tobacco produced metric tons	Cigarettes exports millions	Cigarettes imports millions	Tobacco leaf exports metric tons	Tobacco leaf imports metric tons
Afghanistan	–	–	–	–	1,500	–	–
Albania	7,300	0.88%	8,000	4,000	–	1,500	34
Algeria	5,700	0.03%	7,153	–	–	–	18,000
Andorra	–	–	–	–	–	–	–
Angola	3,100	0.11%	3,000	–	400	–	180
Antigua and Barbuda	–	–	–	–	–	–	–
Argentina	57,300	0.18%	114,156	2,400	2,400	72,580	6,803
Armenia	2,528	0.04%	4,577	–	2,200	319	2,537
Australia	3,185	0.01%	7,762	4,000	1,600	1,803	14,355
Austria	111	0.01%	230	11,803	1,681	931	10,404
Azerbaijan	7,789	0.51%	17,258	500	3,400	11,870	–
Bahamas	–	–	–	–	–	–	55
Bahrain	–	–	–	–	–	–	40
Bangladesh	31,161	0.44%	35,000	–	400	892	2,839
Barbados	–	–	–	55	20	–	4
Belarus	800	0.01%	1,400	–	4,000	–	10,347
Belgium	*380	0.05%	*1,300	*14,000	*8,200	*16,666	*41,014
Belize	–	–	–	20	155	–	84
Benin	917	0.03%	702	–	500	–	50
Bhutan	110	0.07%	160	–	–	–	4
Bolivia	1,060	0.05%	975	–	–	–	530
Bosnia and Herzegovina	2,000	0.25%	3,600	–	1,000	550	890
Botswana	–	–	–	–	900	56	618
Brazil	309,989	0.45%	578,451	700	–	343,029	2,647
Brunei Darussalam	–	–	–	–	800	–	–
Bulgaria	42,000	0.32%	70,000	8,728	1,000	21,000	7,400
Burkina Faso	800	0.03%	400	–	–	–	590
Burundi	360	0.04%	350	–	–	1	1,084
Cambodia	9,669	0.35%	7,665	–	–	1,051	890
Cameroon	3,400	0.03%	4,700	100	5	220	2,400
Canada	25,000	0.06%	71,000	1,600	396	23,075	3,297
Cape Verde	–	–	–	–	–	–	40
Central African Rep.	600	0.04%	500	–	–	140	350
Chad	145	<0.1%	210	–	55	–	100
Chile	3,508	0.16%	10,521	230	135	915	1,837
China	1,441,147	1.1%	2,563,510	41,566	47,740	131,980	27,018
Colombia	18,250	0.3%	33,216	5,500	13,260	10,217	3,331
Comoros	–	–	–	–	–	–	–
Congo	280	0.19%	100	3	30	–	270
Congo, Dem. Rep.	7,700	0.09%	3,600	–	–	–	680
Cook Islands	–	–	–	–	–	–	–
Costa Rica	108	0.20%	200	–	–	960	890
Côte d'Ivoire	20,000	0.28%	10,000	400	500	70	2,300
Croatia	6,100	0.55%	8,600	5,545	15	5,899	3,032
Cuba	45,785	0.85%	30,562	100	–	6,400	4,000
Cyprus	76	0.05%	374	3,550	–	147	420
Czech Republic	–	0.06%	–	16,500	4,000	761	20,242
Denmark	–	–	–	6,000	2,000	1,550	16,050

* data for Belgium and Luxembourg

mber of rkers	Cigarettes manufactured millions	Malboro or equivalent international brand $US per pack	Local brand	Labour needed to buy a pack of Marlboro or equivalent international brand city	minutes	Tax as a proportion of cigarette price percentages	Tobacco excise tax revenue as a proportion of total tax revenue percentages	Tobacco industry documents on the Legacy website	Countries
0	–	–	–	–	–	–	–	7	Afghanistan
1,946	–	–	–	–	–	70%	–	10	Albania
6,096	–	–	–	–	–	–	–	52	Algeria
–	–	–	–	–	–	–	–	133	Andorra
478	–	–	–	–	–	–	–	15	Angola
–	–	–	–	–	–	–	–	9	Antigua and Barbuda
4,650	39,800	1.70	1.50	Buenos Aires	20.5	70%	4.34%	1,931	Argentina
0	–	–	–	–	–	50%	–	6	Armenia
1,569	32,000	3.46	3.20	Sydney	28.4	65%	3.38%	10,472	Australia
1,756	–	3.31	3.04	Vienna	21.8	73%	0.16%	2,907	Austria
1,751	–	0.88	0.33	–	–	–	–	1	Azerbaijan
0	–	–	–	–	–	–	–	153	Bahamas
0	–	1.32	–	Manama	17.6	–	–	212	Bahrain
2,829	–	1.26	0.83	–	–	30%	–	101	Bangladesh
75	–	–	–	–	–	–	–	45	Barbados
–	–	–	–	–	–	–	–	1	Belarus
4,400	*20,750	2.93	2.93	Brussels	22	75%	–	2,502	Belgium
116	–	–	–	–	–	–	–	5	Belize
–	–	–	–	–	–	–	–	13	Benin
0	–	–	–	–	–	–	–	1	Bhutan
197	–	–	–	–	–	61%	–	140	Bolivia
849	–	–	–	–	–	–	–	2	Bosnia and Herzegovina
0	–	–	–	–	–	–	–	32	Botswana
8,807	175,000	0.85	0.80	Rio de Janeiro / Sao Paulo	21.8 / 17.2	75%	7.37%	2,492	Brazil
–	–	1.70	–	–	–	–	–	48	Brunei Darussalam
5,800	55,400	1.13	–	–	–	42%	3.63%	305	Bulgaria
195	–	–	–	–	–	–	–	11	Burkina Faso
180	–	–	–	–	–	–	–	5	Burundi
2,126	–	0.90	–	–	–	20%	–	8	Cambodia
436	–	1.42	0.99	–	–	–	–	53	Cameroon
4,600	58,000	3.40	2.88	Montreal / Toronto	19.4 / 20.7	51%		11,851	Canada
47	–	–	–	–	–	–	–	1	Cape Verde
–	–	–	–	–	–	–	–	1	Central African Rep.
–	–	–	–	–	–	–	–	38	Chad
535	–	1.69	1.43	Santiago de C.	38.4	70%	4.10%	980	Chile
7,472	1,748,500	1.57	1.40	Shanghai	61.8	38%–40%	2.79%	9,047	China
1,243	–	1.03	0.64	Bogota	24.9	45%	0.91%	647	Colombia
–	–	–	–	–	–	–	–	3	Comoros
194	–	–	–	–	–	–	–	21	Congo
1,243	–	–	–	–	–	–	–	–	Congo, Dem. Rep.
–	–	–	–	–	–	–	–	1	Cook Islands
576	–	0.75	0.75	–	–	75%	1.58%	573	Costa Rica
555	–	0.92	0.71	–	–	–	–	10	Côte d'Ivoire
2,050	–	2.06	1.33	–	–	–	0.82%	62	Croatia
14,970	16,000	–	–	–	–	–	–	142	Cuba
272	–	–	–	–	–	–	–	429	Cyprus
2,000	0	1.42	1.13	–	–	58%	–	355	Czech Republic
1,415	–	4.00	4.00	Copenhagen	23	84%	2.03%	1,681	Denmark

103

Table B The Business of Tobacco

	1 Growing Tobacco			2 Tobacco Trade			
	Land devoted to growing tobacco hectares	Agricultural land devoted to tobacco farming percentage of total	Tobacco produced metric tons	Cigarettes exports millions	Cigarettes imports millions	Tobacco leaf exports metric tons	Tobacco leaf imports metric tons
Djibouti	–	–	–	–	–	–	80
Dominica	–	–	–	–	–	–	30
Dominican Republic	13,250	1.28%	17,229	40	–	14,640	–
East Timor	–	–	–	–	–	–	–
Ecuador	1,725	0.02%	3,461	100	–	883	246
Egypt	–	–	–	1,400	500	–	55,040
El Salvador	600	0.10%	1,100	–	–	84	448
Equatorial Guinea	–	–	–	–	–	–	–
Eritrea	–	–	–	–	–	–	–
Estonia	–	–	–	–	600	–	4
Ethiopia	4,500	0.05%	3,000	–	200	–	200
Fiji	180	0.07%	150	12	14	–	130
Finland	–	–	–	193	1,700	1,307	3,904
France	9,254	0.05%	25,534	23,300	67,571	46,023	70,528
Gabon	–	–	–	–	–	–	100
Gambia	–	–	–	–	–	116	793
Georgia	1,801	0.11%	1,855	–	1,500	–	2,000
Germany	3,000	0.03%	8,500	90,637	33,604	41,430	189,669
Ghana	4,200	0.06%	2,500	–	35	255	56
Greece	62,917	1.65%	136,593	17,000	11,000	100,889	19,554
Grenada	–	–	–	–	–	–	30
Guatemala	8,374	0.43%	18,630	1,900	600	9,043	643
Guinea	2,000	0.13%	1,800	–	20	–	70
Guinea-Bissau	–	–	–	–	–	–	–
Guyana	100	0.02%	90	–	–	–	–
Haiti	400	0.05%	550	–	20	–	660
Honduras	11,214	0.47%	4,318	236	–	2,547	3,205
Hungary	5,764	0.14%	10,485	3,500	500	759	17,539
Iceland	–	–	–	–	600	–	–
India	463,200	0.23%	701,700	1,500	200	119,643	1,500
Indonesia	223,000	0.72%	145,000	17,500	140	37,097	40,913
Iran, Isl. Rep.	20,000	0.07%	21,000	–	8,000	1,516	842
Iraq	2,400	0.04%	2,250	–	–	–	2,400
Ireland	–	–	–	2,000	450	83	5,650
Israel	–	0.05%	–	200	2,400	10	4,700
Italy	46,900	0.46%	132,200	193	56,475	93,862	38,830
Jamaica	1,175	0.44%	1,800	40	1,780	130	450
Japan	23,991	0.6%	60,803	13,961	83,478	31	98,919
Jordan	3,099	1.06%	2,667	300	200	483	1,400
Kazakhstan	4,500	0.01%	9,000	12,600	3,000	7,521	6,129
Kenya	4,500	0.19%	7,000	550	50	4,423	50
Kiribati	–	–	–	–	–	–	–
Korea, Republic of	24,300	1.62%	68,198	6,712	9,378	5,618	12,781
Korea, Dem. People's Rep. of	44,000	2.10%	63,000	–	–	5,000	576
Kuwait	–	–	–	–	1,000	–	–
Kyrgyzstan	14,465	0.64%	34,613	–	1,000	35,000	6
Lao People's Dem. Rep.	6,700	0.87%	33,400	–	–	–	260
Latvia	–	–	–	–	1,000	–	1,544

Number of workers	Cigarettes manufactured millions	Malboro or equivalent international brand	Local brand	Labour needed to buy a pack of Marlboro or equivalent international brand — city	minutes	Tax as a proportion of cigarette price percentages	Tobacco excise tax revenue as a proportion of total tax revenue percentages	Tobacco industry documents on the Legacy website	
3 Manufacturing		**4 Costs**				**5 Tax**		**6**	
–	–	–	–	–	–	–	–	29	Djibouti
–	–	–	–	–	–	–	–	35	Dominica
1,480	–	–	–	–	–	–	–	239	Dominican Republic
–	–	–	–	–	–	–	–	–	East Timor
361	–	1.90	1.30	–	–	–	–	617	Ecuador
7,469	40,000	1.16	1.16	–	–	57%	1.34%	629	Egypt
0	–	–	–	–	–	42%	–	310	El Salvador
–	–	–	–	–	–	–	–	0	Equatorial Guinea
–	–	–	–	–	–	–	–	1	Eritrea
–	–	–	–	–	–	70%	1.29%	20	Estonia
898	–	–	–	–	–	–	–	9	Ethiopia
98	–	–	–	–	–	–	–	58	Fiji
700	–	3.73	3.35	Helsinki	28.7	73%	2.03%	4,856	Finland
4,400	48,000	3.13	2.75	Paris	20.5	75%	0.37%	5,298	France
50	–	1.32	1.22	–	–	–	–	16	Gabon
0	–	–	–	–	–	–	–	18	Gambia
–	–	1.00	–	–	–	–	–	1,732	Georgia
5,455	205,500	2.81	2.75	Berlin Frankfurt	18.4 17.3	72%	1.38%	9,489	Germany
1,121	–	1.40	–	–	–	–	–	40	Ghana
9,943	28,200	2.05	1.64	Athens	24	73%	8.69%	1,228	Greece
19	–	–	–	–	–	–	–	18	Grenada
556	–	1.29	0.97	–	–	–	–	628	Guatemala
–	–	–	–	–	–	–	–	2,025	Guinea
–	–	–	–	–	–	–	–	3	Guinea-Bissau
193	–	–	–	–	–	–	–	22	Guyana
350	–	–	–	–	–	–	–	87	Haiti
–	–	–	–	–	–	–	–	163	Honduras
2,750	30,000	1.09	0.77	Budapest	71.4	42%	0.02%	480	Hungary
–	–	4.43	4.53	–	–	–	–	235	Iceland
37,692	90,000	1.24	0.91	Mumbai	102.5	75%	2.43%	1,447	India
37,401	190,000	0.62	0.62	Jakarta	61.7	30%	3.38%	834	Indonesia
7,197	–	0.96	0.46	–	–	–	–	289	Iran, Isl. Rep.
1,000	–	–	–	–	–	–	–	129	Iraq
1,279	–	4.47	4.47	Dublin	30.6	75%	–	6,605	Ireland
600	–	3.22	1.91	Tel Aviv	29.3	–	–	3,277	Israel
3,330	55,300	2.70	1.93	Milan	26	73%	–	2,165	Italy
750	–	–	–	–	–	42%	–	227	Jamaica
14,200	265,000	2.34	2.09	Tokyo	8.9	60%	0.02%	17,611	Japan
1,051	–	2.04	0.98	–	–	–	–	5,954	Jordan
–	–	–	–	–	–	–	–	33	Kazakhstan
1,701	–	1.55	0.90	Nairobi	157.6	–	0.09%	169	Kenya
–	–	–	–	–	–	–	–	0	Kiribati
3,600	84,600	1.50	1.26	Seoul	26.6	60%	3.46%	***1,717	Korea, Republic of
–	–	–	–	–	–	–	–	***1,717	Korea, Dem. People's Rep. of
0	–	1.10	–	–	–	–	–	571	Kuwait
1,294	–	–	–	–	–	–	–	1	Kyrgyzstan
500	–	–	–	–	–	–	–	30	Lao People's Dem. Rep.
286	–	–	–	–	–	–	–	13	Latvia

**combined total for Democratic People's Republic of Korea and Republic of Korea

Table B The Business of Tobacco

Countries	1 Growing Tobacco			2 Tobacco Trade			
	Land devoted to growing tobacco hectares	Agricultural land devoted to tobacco farming percentage of total	Tobacco produced metric tons	Cigarettes exports millions	Cigarettes imports millions	Tobacco leaf exports metric tons	Tobacco leaf imports metric ton
Lebanon	9,700	2.02%	13,500	–	1,400	3,100	270
Lesotho	–	–	–	–	–	–	–
Liberia	–	–	–	–	200	–	–
Libyan Arab Jamahiriya	650	0.03%	1,500	–	2,200	–	3,100
Lithuania	–	–	–	–	1,500	–	2,915
Luxembourg	*380	–	*1,300	*14,000	*8,200	*16,666	*41,014
Macedonia, Former Yugos. Rep. of	25,000	1.66%	32,000	–	500	9,900	2,200
Madagascar	2,110	0.11%	2,000	–	1	40	362
Malawi	113,823	6.18%	120,000	30	80	93,000	800
Malaysia	12,500	0.14%	7,260	10,609	1,037	274	19,974
Maldives	–	–	–	–	–	–	70
Mali	230	0.02%	180	–	–	–	60
Malta	–	–	–	250	50	1	7
Marshall Islands	–	–	–	–	–	–	–
Mauritania	–	–	–	–	–	–	800
Mauritius	440	0.63%	700	–	–	–	89
Mexico	22,674	0.06%	45,205	20	5	10,509	8,623
Micronesia, Federated States of	–	–	–	–	–	–	–
Moldova, Republic of	18,608	0.92%	22,407	5,300	400	21,811	2.652
Monaco	–	–	–	–	–	–	–
Mongolia	–	–	–	–	–	–	–
Morocco	3,500	0.03%	3,500	–	3,100	–	8,021
Mozambique	7,000	0.08%	9,470	–	40	–	600
Myanmar	30,000	0.31%	46,260	800	800	–	622
Namibia	–	–	–	–	–	–	–
Nauru	–	–	–	–	–	–	–
Nepal	4,283	0.20%	3,809	–	–	–	3,100
Netherlands	–	–	–	101,550	14,725	19,630	112,607
New Zealand	–	–	–	75	20	36	3,930
Nicaragua	1,395	0.05%	2,000	–	–	1,243	775
Niger	1,000	0.03%	850	–	800	413	100
Nigeria	22,000	0.07%	9,200	–	8,500	180	1,500
Niue	–	–	–	–	–	–	–
Norway	–	–	–	50	1,000	364	6,480
Oman	270	0.18%	1,300	–	–	514	327
Pakistan	56,400	0.22%	107,700	400	4,000	2,446	180
Palau	–	–	–	–	–	–	–
Panama	1,100	0.17%	1,800	–	100	152	2
Papua New Guinea	–	–	–	–	5	–	140
Paraguay	7,000	0.2%	11,000	2,500	2,500	4,625	5,500
Peru	13,500	0.06%	17,231	–	10	144	628
Philippines	40,869	0.59%	49,493	3,105	2,614	17,639	26.790
Poland	14,057	0.13%	29,545	7,716	104	4,955	60,288
Portugal	2,132	0.07%	6,193	3,800	1,606	3,505	7,840
Qatar	–	–	–	–	–	–	20
Romania	10,970	0.1%	14,800	–	5,500	838	25,257
Russian Federation	1,700	<0.1%	1,600	900	15,000	420	263,129
Rwanda	2,800	0.24%	3,800	–	30	–	30

Sources: see page 124

* data for Belgium and Luxembou

3 Manufacturing		4 Costs				5 Tax		6	Countries
umber of orkers	Cigarettes manufactured millions	Malboro or equivalent international brand $US per pack	Local brand	Labour needed to buy a pack of Marlboro or equivalent international brand — city	minutes	Tax as a proportion of cigarette price percentages	Tobacco excise tax revenue as a proportion of total tax revenue percentages	Tobacco industry documents on the Legacy website	
3,800	–	–	–	–	–	–	–	610	Lebanon
–	–	–	–	–	–	–	–	6	Lesotho
91	–	–	–	–	–	–	–	105	Liberia
1,251	–	4.55	1.82	–	–	–	–	24	Libyan Arab Jamahiriya
418	–	–	–	–	–	–	0.16%	44	Lithuania
–	*20,750	2.24	1.90	Luxembourg	12	–	–	495	Luxembourg
5,604	–	–	–	–	–	–	–	24	Macedonia, Former Yugos. Rep. of
814	–	–	–	–	–	–	–	14	Madagascar
74	–	–	–	–	–	–	–	421	Malawi
9,873	–	1.13	1.08	Kuala Lumpur	20.7	33%	–	1,429	Malaysia
–	–	–	–	–	–	–	–	3	Maldives
–	–	–	–	–	–	–	–	31	Mali
158	–	–	–	–	–	–	–	140	Malta
–	–	–	–	–	–	–	–	–	Marshall Islands
–	–	–	–	–	–	–	–	–	Mauritania
207	–	–	–	–	–	–	–	60	Mauritius
5,122	46,500	1.55	1.24	Mexico City	49.4	60%	1.41%	2,121	Mexico
–	–	–	–	–	–	–	–	2	Micronesia, Federated States of
–	–	1	–	–	–	–	–	2	Moldova, Republic of
–	–	–	–	–	–	–	–	767	Monaco
0	–	–	–	–	–	–	–	8	Mongolia
2,301	–	2.63	1.36	–	–	–	–	179	Morocco
–	–	–	–	–	–	–	–	32	Mozambique
2,059	–	–	–	–	–	–	–	440	Myanmar
0	–	–	–	–	–	–	–	1	Namibia
–	–	–	–	–	–	–	–	1	Nauru
3,142	–	–	–	–	–	73%	6.37%	39	Nepal
4,739	90,000	2.80	2.56	Amsterdam	18.5	72%	1.44%	1,956	Netherlands
450	–	3.71	3.69	Auckland	35.3	68%	–	2,353	New Zealand
–	–	–	–	–	–	–	–	82	Nicaragua
–	–	–	–	–	–	–	–	29	Niger
0	–	0.86	0.86	–	–	–	–	529	Nigeria
–	–	–	–	–	–	–	–	1	Niue
–	–	6.48	6.48	Oslo	38.5	78%	1.76%	2,755	Norway
0	–	–	–	–	–	–	–	87	Oman
5,701	36,644	0.83	0.53	–	–	73%	0.11%	634	Pakistan
–	–	–	–	–	–	–	–	5	Palau
177	–	1.20	1.20	Panama	81.4	–	–	1,220	Panama
617	–	1.85	1.85	–	–	–	–	60	Papua New Guinea
250	–	1.10	0.93	–	–	–	–	168	Paraguay
470	–	1.42	1.34	–	–	–	–	440	Peru
14,682	74,400	0.67	0.51	Manila	41.8	63%	–	1,907	Philippines
12,440	110,000	1.51	1.13	Warsaw	55.7	39%	3.26%	2,169	Poland
1,193	–	1.86	1.77	Lisbon	26.2	81%	–	495	Portugal
–	–	–	–	–	–	–	–	101	Qatar
7,500	21,000	1.01	0.88	–	–	–	0.20%	90	Romania
17,600	**293,000	0.98	0.59	Moscow	71.3	–	–	503	Russian Federation
0	–	–	–	–	–	–	–	1	Rwanda

* data for Former Soviet Union

Table B The Business of Tobacco

Countries	1 Growing Tobacco			2 Tobacco Trade			
	Land devoted to growing tobacco hectares	Agricultural land devoted to tobacco farming percentage of total	Tobacco produced metric tons	Cigarettes exports millions	Cigarettes imports millions	Tobacco leaf exports metric tons	Tobacco leaf import metric to
Saint Kitts and Nevis	–	–	–	–	–	–	–
Saint Lucia	–	–	–	–	–	–	20
Saint Vincent and Grenadines	70	0.55%	85	–	–	–	30
Samoa	40	0.03%	135	3,250	25	–	–
San Marino	–	–	–	–	–	–	–
Sao Tome and Principe	–	–	–	–	–	–	–
Saudi Arabia	–	–	–	150	20,000	2	622
Senegal	–	–	–	3	500	366	1,647
Seychelles	–	–	–	–	15	–	40
Sierra Leone	40	0.11%	20	200	13	100	500
Singapore	–	0.30%	–	58,745	49,350	2,266	12,158
Slovakia	1,134	0.47%	1,870	50	900	1,775	5,674
Slovenia	–	–	–	–	–	750	8,500
Solomon Islands	100	0.16%	85	–	25	–	20
Somalia	250	0.02%	100	–	–	–	130
South Africa	14,100	0.09%	29,700	1,926	324	15,905	6,930
Spain	13,450	0.09%	42,250	5,133	25,175	25,615	53,895
Sri Lanka	4,780	0.45%	6,000	400	50	2,374	3,825
Sudan	–	–	–	–	700	–	70
Suriname	–	–	–	–	20	–	420
Swaziland	194	0.04%	71	–	–	2	7
Sweden	–	–	–	400	2,000	1,653	10,789
Switzerland	651	0.17%	1,182	23,400	200	7,372	31,486
Syrian Arab Republic	16,726	0.25%	26,112	500	2,000	2,315	–
Tajikistan	5,200	0.54%	13,500	–	1,000	–	7,000
Tanzania, United Republic of	40,000	1.06%	26,670	12,265	–	21,350	250
Thailand	51,800	0.21%	74,200	1,500	8,000	25,025	10,177
Togo	4,000	0.16%	2,000	–	1,000	–	3
Tonga	–	–	–	–	–	–	–
Trinidad and Tobago	–	0.04%	–	–	2	–	2,065
Tunisia	3,100	0.08%	3,400	–	2,000	278	8,013
Turkey	290,000	0.77%	260,000	111,006	30	129,284	48,846
Turkmenistan	800	0.07%	2,000	–	1,500	–	800
Tuvalu	–	–	–	–	–	–	–
Uganda	7,500	0.11%	10,000	–	–	4,714	144
Ukraine	4,300	0.02%	3,000	–	20,000	1,579	70,000
United Arab Emirates	50	0.07%	608	–	8,000	60	236
United Kingdom of Gr. Br. & N Ir.	–	–	–	2	45,018	9,945	128,569
United States of America	191,176	0.15%	477,630	148,261	15,064	190,538	241,062
Uruguay	830	0.06%	2,800	22,950	40	74	8,954
Uzbekistan	10,500	0.17%	19,000	15	7,500	–	5,450
Vanuatu	–	–	–	–	–	–	–
Venezuela	6,000	0.23%	11,288	250	50	186	10,507
Viet Nam	24,400	0.41%	27,200	–	2,000	96	16,000
Yemen	5,209	0.26%	12,581	2,000	150	14	8,502
Yugoslavia	9,858	0.26%	11,341	3,250	14,500	3,710	2,700
Zambia	2,900	0.06%	3,200	–	–	3,600	1,100
Zimbabwe	90,769	2.56%	227,726	2,000	–	163,933	6,723

108   Sources: see page 124

3 Manufacturing		4 Costs				5 Tax		6	
Number of workers	Cigarettes manufactured millions	Malboro or equivalent international brand $US per pack	Local brand	Labour needed to buy a pack of Marlboro or equivalent international brand city	minutes	Tax as a proportion of cigarette price percentages	Tobacco excise tax revenue as a proportion of total tax revenue percentages	Tobacco industry documents on the Legacy website	Countries
–	–	–	–	–	–	–	–	14	Saint Kitts and Nevis
0	–	–	–	–	–	–	–	10	Saint Lucia
20	–	–	–	–	–	–	–	362	Saint Vincent and Grenadines
0	–	–	–	–	–	–	–	7	Samoa
–	–	–	–	–	–	–	3.35%	5	San Marino
–	–	–	–	–	–	–	–	27	Sao Tome and Principe
–	–	1.30	0.93	–	–	–	–	1,806	Saudi Arabia
400	–	0.71	0.28	–	–	–	–	89	Senegal
–	–	–	–	–	–	44%	3.71%	14	Seychelles
194	–	–	–	–	–	–	–	27	Sierra Leone
0	–	3.92	3.52	Singapore	42.6	–	–	1,969	Singapore
0	–	–	–	–	–	34%	–	17	Slovakia
–	–	–	–	–	–	63%	–	36	Slovenia
–	–	–	–	–	–	–	–	7	Solomon Islands
526	–	–	–	–	–	–	–	65	Somalia
3,110	37,795	1.34	1.34	Johannesburg	19.5	33%	1.15%	624	South Africa
9,277	79,000	2.16	1.15	Barcelona Madrid	21.1 21.4	72%	2.37%	3,183	Spain
23,114	–	1.78	1.66	–	–	24%	–	66	Sri Lanka
497	–	–	–	–	–	–	–	87	Sudan
80	–	–	–	–	–	–	–	17	Suriname
0	–	–	–	–	–	–	–	21	Swaziland
560	–	3.75	3.64	Stockholm	27.6	69%	1.63%	3,512	Sweden
–	39,515	2.80	2.80	Geneva Zurich	12.5 11.1	52%	1.69%	4,734	Switzerland
–	–	1.12	0.56	–	–	–	–	71	Syrian Arab Republic
–	–	–	–	–	–	–	–	1	Tajikistan
4,551	–	–	–	–	–	–	–	53	Tanzania, United Republic of
4,033	47,000	1.08	0.69	Bangkok	35	62%	–	1,240	Thailand
–	–	–	–	–	–	–	–	23	Togo
0	–	–	–	–	–	–	–	4	Tonga
166	–	–	–	–	–	–	–	157	Trinidad and Tobago
3,554	–	1.96	–	–	–	–	–	65	Tunisia
1,504	–	1.23	0.89	Istanbul	30	42%	0.21%	1,033	Turkey
–	–	–	–	–	–	–	–	0	Turkmenistan
–	–	–	–	–	–	–	–	0	Tuvalu
719	–	1.89	–	–	–	–	–	33	Uganda
7,000	–	0.80	–	–	–	–	–	29	Ukraine
0	–	1.77	0.29	Abu Dhabi	19.7	–	–	144	United Arab Emirates
6,450	114,300	6.24	6.25	London	39.7	78%	3.23%	9,181	United Kingdom of Gr. Br. & N Ir.
7,300	716,500	3.71	3.60	Chicago Los Angeles	18 20	24%	0.44%	78,615	United States of America
396	–	3.14	1.42	–	–	60%	2.64%	300	Uruguay
–	–	–	1.11	–	–	–	–	29	Uzbekistan
–	–	–	–	–	–	–	–	0	Vanuatu
2,581	–	1.42	1.28	Caracas	28.5	50%	2.30%	1,145	Venezuela
–	–	0.72	0.57	–	–	36%	–	329	Viet Nam
961	–	–	–	–	–	–	–	28	Yemen
4,900	0	0.94	0.28	–	–	–	–	522	Yugoslavia
503	–	2.03	–	–	–	30%	0.04%	73	Zambia
4,290	–	1.15	0.65	–	–	80%	1.17%	864	Zimbabwe

109

GLOSSARY OF TERMS USED IN *THE TOBACCO ATLAS*

Advertising – Any commercial effort to promote, including the use of sponsorship activities, the use, image or awareness of a tobacco product, its trade marks, brand name or manufacturer.

Areca nut – The fruit of the Areca Catechu tree. Areca nut is commonly combined with betel leaves, slaked lime, and tobacco and chewed as betel-quid, particularly in areas of Southeast Asia. In Northeast India, the use of fermented areca nut (tamol) is common.

Betel-quid – A mixture which typically consists of areca nut, tobacco, slaked lime and sweetening or flavouring agents, wrapped in a betel leaf. Betel-quid is chewed in many countries in Asia, such as India, Sri Lanka, Bangladesh, Cambodia and Malaysia.

Bidis – Consist of a small amount of tobacco, hand-wrapped in dried temburni leaf and tied with string. Despite their small size, their tar and carbon monoxide deliveries can be higher than manufactured cigarettes because of the need to puff harder to keep bidis lit. Bidis are used extensively in areas of Southeast Asia and are the most commonly smoked tobacco product in India.

Chilum – A straight, conical pipe made of clay. Chilum smoking is practiced mostly among males in the northern rural areas of India. The pipe is held vertically, and to prevent the tobacco from entering the mouth, a pebble or stopper is inserted into the top of the chilum. The entire pipe is usually filled with tobacco, and the mouth-piece is wrapped with a wet piece of cloth to protect the mouth from the heat and to serve as a filter.

Cigars – Made of air-cured and fermented tobaccos with a tobacco wrapper, they come in many shapes and sizes, from cigarette-sized cigarillos, double coronas, cheroots, stumpen, chuttas and dhumtis. In reverse chutta and dhumti smoking the ignited end of the cigar is placed inside the mouth.

Clove cigarettes – *see* **Kreteks**

Consumption – Total cigarette consumption is the number of cigarettes sold annually in a country, usually in millions of sticks. Total cigarette consumption is

calculated by adding a country's cigarette production and imports and subtracting exports. "Per adult" cigarette consumption is calculated by dividing total cigarette consumption by the total population of those who are 15 years and older. Smuggling may account for inaccuracies in these estimates.

Excess mortality – The amount by which death rates for a given population group (e.g. smokers) exceed that of another population group chosen as a reference or standard (e.g. non-smokers).

Health warnings – Verbal, written or visual warnings, required by governments on packets or advertisements of all tobacco products.

Hookah – *see* **Water pipe**

Ingredients – Every component of the product that is smoked or chewed, including all additives and flavourings, contents such as paper, ink and filters, and materials used in the manufacturing process (such as adhesives etc.) present in the finished product in burnt or unburned form, and whether the tobacco has been genetically modified.

Kreteks – Clove-flavoured cigarettes. They contain a wide range of exotic flavourings and eugenol, which has an anaesthetising effect, allowing for greater and deeper inhalation.

Manufactured cigarettes – Consist of shredded or reconstituted tobacco, processed with hundreds of chemicals, wrapped in paper, and often with a filter and manufactured by a machine. They are the predominant form of tobacco used worldwide.

Nicotine – nicotinic alkaloids.

Nicotine replacement therapy (NRT) – A type of pharmacological treatment used as an aid to smoking cessation. It includes devices such as transdermal patches, nicotine gum, nicotine nasal sprays and inhalers.

Pan masala – Pan masala or betel quid consists of four main ingredients: tobacco, areca nuts and slaked lime wrapped in a betel leaf. It can also contain other

110

sweetenings and flavouring agents. Varieties of pan include kaddipudi, hogesoppu, gundi, kadapam, zarda, pattiwala, kiwam, mishri, and pills. It is commonly chewed in parts of Southeast Asia, especially in rural India.

Passive smoking – Inhaling cigarette, cigar, or pipe smoke produced by another individual. It is composed of second-hand smoke (exhaled by the smoker), and sidestream smoke (which drifts off the tip of the cigarette or cigar or pipe bowl).

Pipes – Made of briar, slate, clay or other substance. Tobacco is placed in a bowl and smoke is inhaled through the stem, sometimes through water.

Prevalence – Smoking prevalence is the percentage of smokers in the total population. Adult smoking is usually defined as aged 15 years and above.

Promotion – A representation about a product or service by any means, whether directly or indirectly, including any communication of information about a product or service and its price and distribution, that is likely to influence and shape attitudes, beliefs and behaviours about the product or service.

Retailer – A person who is engaged in a business that includes the sale of a tobacco product to consumers.

Risk – The likelihood of incurring a particular event or circumstance (e.g. risk of disease measures the chances of an individual contracting a disease).

Smoke-free areas – Areas where smoking or holding a lighted cigarette, cigar or pipe is banned.

Smoker – Someone who, at the time of the survey, smokes any tobacco product either daily or occasionally.

Snuff – Moist snuff is taken orally. A small amount of ground tobacco is held in the mouth between the cheek and gum. Increasingly, manufacturers are pre-packaging moist snuff into small paper or cloth packets to make use of the product easier and neater. Other products include khaini, shammaah, nass/naswa. Dry snuff is powdered tobacco that is inhaled through the nasal passages or taken orally.

Tar – The raw anhydrous nicotine-free condensate of smoke.

Tar and nicotine yield – The amount of tar and nicotine in milligrams in one cigarette, as determined by a machine designed to measure smoke. Machine yields of tar and nicotine levels are not necessarily what smokers actually inhale.

Tobacco attributable health care costs – Health costs calculated on the average proportion of particular diseases attributable to tobacco use.
Direct costs include: costs related to the average proportion of the occurrence of disease attributable to tobacco; health services costs such as hospital services, physician and outpatient services, prescription drugs, nursing home services, home healthcare, allied healthcare; changed expenditures from increased utilisation of services.
Indirect costs include: costs imposed on a household from tobacco-related illness or premature death; loss of production and earnings; household health; psychological costs, such as the effects of grief.

Tobacco attributable mortality – The number of deaths attributable to tobacco use within a specific population.

Tobacco control organisation – A non-profit organisation whose purpose is to reduce tobacco consumption and protect nonsmokers from the effects of involuntary smoking.

Tobacco industry documents – Previously secret, internal industry papers that have now been placed in the public domain as a result of court rulings.

Tobacco taxes – Taxes levied on tobacco products. There are two basic methods of tobacco taxation:
• nominal or specific taxes – taxes based on a set amount of tax per cigarette or gram of tobacco.
• *Ad valorem* taxes – taxes assessed as a percentage mark-up on the retail selling price of tobacco products.
Total tobacco tax refers to a combination of both methods plus any value added tax (VAT) where applicable.

Tobacco product – Any product manufactured wholly or partly from tobacco and intended for use by smoking, inhalation, chewing, sniffing or sucking, with the exception of medicinal preparations containing nicotine.

Tobacco production – Tobacco leaf production in metric tons refers to the actual tobacco leaves harvested from the field, excluding harvesting and threshing losses and any part of the tobacco crop not harvested for any reason.

Tobacco use – The consumption of tobacco products by burning, chewing, inhalation, or other forms of ingestion.

Water pipe – A water pipe, or hookah, consists of a receptacle for water which has an opening on the top to which a long wooden stem is fixed, the lower end being below water level. At the top of this stem, a small bowl is attached for tobacco. The tobacco is drawn through the water and inhaled through a long tube fixed to an outlet on the side of the receptacle. Cut, shredded tobacco moistened with molasses or other sweeteners, is kept in the bowl and burned with charcoal.

1 The History of Tobacco

Encyclopaedia Britannica, 1888, Vol XXIV: 423–427

Historical Background: A Chronology. Duke University - The Tobacco Project, 4 November 2000

Jelbert H, *Tobacco – A brief history*, Health Education Authority, UK, July 1996

Kluger R, *Ashes to Ashes: America's Hundred-Year War, the Public Health and the Unabashed Triumph of Philip Morris*, Alfred A Knopf, New York, 1996

Moyer DB, *The Tobacco Almanac: A reference book of fact, figures, quotations about tobacco*, October 1998 (self published)

Routh HB, Bhowmik KR, Parish JL, Parish LC. *Historical Aspects of Tobacco Use and Smoking*. Clinics in Dermatology 1998, 16(5):539–544

U.S. Department of Health and Human Services, *Smoking and Health in the Americas*, A 1992 Report of the Surgeon General, in collaboration with the Pan American Health Organization, 1992

Walton J (ed), *The Faber Book of Smoking*, Faber and Faber, London, 2000

Tobacco milestones: A brief history of tobacco, adapted from a chronology by the National Clearinghouse on Tobacco and Health, Ottawa, Canada, 1996

Yach D, Saloojee Y, McIntyre D, *Smoking in South Africa: Health and Economic Impact*, MRC, Cape Town, South Africa, 1992

Part One:
PREVALENCE AND HEALTH

2 Types of Tobacco Use

MAIN MAP

Gupta PC. Survey of socio-demographic characteristics of tobacco use among 99,598 individuals in Bombay, India using hand-held computers, *Tobacco Control 1996*; 5(2): 114–120

World Health Organization. *Tobacco or Health: A Global Status Report*. Geneva, Switzerland, WHO, 1997

World Health Organization, *Guidelines for controlling and monitoring the tobacco epidemic*, Geneva, Switzerland, WHO, 1998

3 Male Smoking

MAIN MAP

Albania Current tobacco smoking; World Health Organization Regional Office for Europe (2001). The European Tobacco Control Report: review of implementation of the Third Action Plan for a Tobacco Free Europe 1997–2001 Copenhagen

Algeria Current tobacco smoking in Setif area; information provided by Hamdi Cherif Mokhtar, Hospital Mere Enfant. 1997–98

Andorra Regular daily smoking; WHO Regional Office for Europe. (2000). Health for all statistical database. Copenhagen

Argentina Current smoking among the urban population; Rojas, M <rojasmar@paho.org> (June 19 2000). Re: Smoking prevalence in Latin America. [data transfer via email]

Armenia Current tobacco smoking; World Health Organization Regional Office for Europe (2001). The European Tobacco Control Report: review of implementation of the Third Action Plan for a Tobacco Free Europe 1997–2001 Copenhagen.

Australia 2001 National Drug Strategy Household Survey (Daily Smoking), May 2002, Australian Institute of Health and Welfare

Austria Regular smoking measured by Statistik Austria, Microcensus. 1997

Azerbaijan Daily smoking based on household budget research results; Azerbaijan's central statistics institute, 'AZSTAT' azstat@azeri.com. 1999

Bahamas Regular smoking measured by the Ministry of Health; WHO (1997). Tobacco or health: a global status report Geneva.

Bahrain Hamadeh RR. Smoking in Gulf Countries. *Bahrain Medical Bulletin*1998; 20(3): 91–4. As reported in Eastern Mediterranean Tobacco Control Profile (survey 2002)

Bangladesh SEAR Country Profiles, 2002

Barbados 1993 Risk Factor Survey conducted by the Barbados Ministry of Health and the Pan American Health Organization

Belarus Daily cigarette smoking; information provided by Dr. S Novoselova, Head, Department of Households Sample Surveys, Ministry of Statistics and Analysis of the Republic of Belarus, 1999

Belgium Daily cigarette smoking measured by Le Centre de Recherche et d'Information des Organisations de Consommateurs (CRIOC-SOBEMAP); information provided by Luk Joossens. 2000

Benin Current smoking of 20 cigarettes per day in the city of Cotonou (1988 is date of publication); Fourn, L & Monteiro, B (1988). Smoking and health in Benin. World Health Forum, 9, 589–590

Bolivia Current smoking among the urban population, Rojas, M <rojasmar@paho.org> (2000, June 19). Re: Smoking prevalence in Latin America. [data transfer via email].

Bosnia and Herzegovina Regular daily smoking measured by the Public Health Institute; WHO Regional Office for Europe (2000). Health for all statistical database, Copenhagen

Botswana Smoking measured by a national health status evaluation programme; WHO. (1997). Tobacco or health: a global status report, Geneva

Brazil Current cigarette smoking; ERC Statistics International (1998). The World Cigarette Market, Suffolk, Great Britain.

Brunei Darussalam Regular cigarette smoking in Tutong town (third largest town in Brunei), (1979 is date of publication); Woodcock, A (1979). Smoking in Tutong, Brunei: a changing habit, *Med J Malaysia*, XXXIV (1), 3–5. Adult smoking prevalence was estimated at 20%; WHO (1997). Tobacco or health: a global status report, Geneva

Bulgaria Regular smoking (1–5 cigarettes daily, every day); Baev, S (1997). Health Status of the Population (Statistics 3, 1997) Sofia: National Statistical Institute

Cambodia 1999 ADRA TOH KAP survey (urban Phnom Penh), as reported in the WPRO Country Profiles, 2000

Cameroon Current smoking; Cameroon smoking population (2000). TMA-International Tobacco Guide (ITG). [CD-ROM] Tobacco Information Service

Canada Current tobacco smoking (smoking at the time of the interview, includes daily and occasional smoking); Health Canada. 1. Summary of Results. Canadian Tobacco Use Monitoring Survey, Wave 1, February–June 1999

Chad Current cigarette smoking in Sahr (third largest city in Chad); Leonard, L (1996). Cigarette smoking and perceptions about smoking and health in Chad, *East Afr Med J*, 73(8), 509–512

Chile Daily tobacco smoking in the three months prior to the survey; Departmento Informacion Social Mideplan. (1998). Prevalencia de tabaquismo Chile (Casen)

China 1996 National Survey of Smoking Prevalence, as reported in the WPRO Country Profiles, 2000

Colombia Current smoking; Rojas, M. <rojasmar@paho.org> (19 June 2000). Re: Smoking prevalence in Latin America. [data transfer via email]

Cook Islands Regular smoking (at least one cigarette per day) among Polynesians in Cook Islands-Rarotonga, Li, N. et al. (1994). Prevalence of coronary heart disease indicated by electrocardiogram abnormalities and risk factors in developing countries. *J Clin Epidemiol*, 47(6), 599–611

Costa Rica Current smoking; Rojas, M <rojasmar@paho.org> (19 June 2000). Re: Smoking prevalence in Latin America. [data transfer via email]

Cote d'Ivoire Current cigarette smoking in Abidjan, Schmidt, D et al. (1981). En quete sur la consommation tabagique en milieu africain a Abidjan, Poumon-Coeur, 37, 87–94; WHO Tobacco or Health program estimated that 20–40% of males and 1–2% of females smoked in 1993 (Dr. J R Menchaca)

Croatia Current tobacco smoking; World Health Organization Regional Office for Europe (2001). The European Tobacco Control Report: review of implementation of the Third Action Plan for a Tobacco Free Europe 1997–2001, Copenhagen

Cuba Current smoking of at least one cigarette per day at the time of the survey; Perez, P V et al. (1995). National survey in risk factors. Havana: National Institute for Hygiene, Epidemiology and Microbiology, Ministry of Health and National Statistic Office.

Cyprus Survey on Tobacco Prevalence in Cyprus, 1998, as reported in Eastern Mediterranean Tobacco Control Profile (survey 2002)

Czech Republic Current tobacco smoking, World Health Organization Regional Office for Europe (2001). The European Tobacco Control Report: review of implementation of the Third Action Plan for a Tobacco Free Europe 1997–2001, Copenhagen

Dem. Rep. of the Congo Active tobacco smoking ("do you consume tobacco") in Kinshasa City; convenience sample of 330 women and 218 men, mean age = 20.73; Abraham, M B et al. (1998). Rapport sur l'analyse de la situation actuelle du tabagisme en Republique Democratique du Congo, Organisation Mondiale de la Sante

Denmark Current tobacco smoking; World Health Organization Regional Office for Europe. (2001). The European Tobacco Control Report: review of implementation of the Third Action Plan for a Tobacco Free Europe 1997–2001, Copenhagen

Djibouti Survey on nutritional status in Djibouti, 1995, as reported in Eastern Mediterranean Tobacco Control Profile (survey 2002)

Dominican Republic Current cigarette smoking; Aono, H et al. (1997). Prevalence of risk factors for coronary heart disease among Dominicans in the Dominican Republic: comparison with Japanese and Americans using existing data. *J Epidemiol*, 7(4), 238–243

Ecuador Current cigarette smoking ('Do you smoke cigarettes now?') in Quito and Guayaquil; Ockene, J K et al. (1996). Smoking in Ecuador: prevalence, knowledge, and attitudes, *Tobacco Control*, 5, 121–126; a 1995 study among 12-49 year olds found that 28.3% of the population were current smokers (PAHO)

Egypt National survey of Tobacco, MOH, 1998, as reported in Eastern Mediterranean Tobacco Control Profile (survey 2002)

El Salvador Current smoking in urban areas; Gallup Organization, Inc. (1988). The incidence of smoking in Central and South America. Conducted for the American Cancer Society

Estonia Current tobacco smoking; World Health Organization Regional Office for Europe (2001). The European Tobacco Control Report: review of implementation of the Third Action Plan for a Tobacco Free Europe 1997–2001, Copenhagen

Ethiopia Tobacco use; Selassie, A G et al. (1996). Rapid assessment of drug abuse in Ethiopia, *Bull Narc*, 83 (1&2), 53–63

Fiji Current smoking; Maxwell, J C (1998). The Maxwell Consumer Report: international tobacco report – parts one and two. Richmond, Virginia: Davenport & Company LLC

Finland Daily cigarette and pipe smoking; National Public Health Institute (1998) Health behaviour among Finnish adult population, Spring 1998. Helsinki: Puska, P et al.

France Current tobacco smoking; Comité français d'éducation pour la santé (2000), Health Barometer 2000

Gambia Current tobacco smoking among urban adults; Walraven, G E, et al. (2001). Asthma, smoking and chronic cough in rural and urban adult communities in The Gambia, *Clinical and Experimental Allergy*, 31(11), 1679–1685

Georgia Current smoking in Tbilisi measured by the Chronic Diseases Center (1999 is the date of publication); Grim, C E et al. (1999). Prevalence of cardiovascular risk factors in the Republic of Georgia, *J Hum Hypertens*, 13, 243–247

Germany Current tobacco smoking; World Health Organization Regional Office for Europe (2001). The European Tobacco Control Report: review of implementation of the Third Action Plan for a Tobacco Free Europe 1997–2001, Copenhagen

Ghana Current smoking in the suburbs of Accra (Sobon-Zongo-Larterbiokorshie area) measured by the Ghana Medical School; information provided by the Health and Humanitarian Environmental Society, 1980

Greece Current tobacco smoking; World Health Organization Regional Office for Europe (2001). The European Tobacco Control Report: review of implementation of the Third Action Plan for a Tobacco Free Europe 1997–2001, Copenhagen

Guatemala Current daily and occasional smoking in urban areas measured by the 1989 National Survey on Smoking; Arango, L (1989). Encuesta nacional de tabaquismo. Comision Nacional de Lucha contra el Tabaco

Guinea Current smoking in five districts of the capital city of Conakry (Dixinn, Kaloum, Matam, Matoto & Ratoma), study does not claim to be representative of the Guinean population (1998 is date of publication); Ngom, A. et al. (1998). Investigation of nicotine addiction in Guinea. Conakry: Department of Health & Office of WHO in Guinea

Haiti Current tobacco use; Narcotics Awareness and Education Project (NAE) (1991). National study of drug prevalence and attitudes toward drug use in Haiti. Haiti: Development Associates, Inc.

Honduras Current smoking in urban areas; Gallup Organization, Inc. (1988). The incidence of smoking in Central and Latin America. Conducted for the American Cancer Society

Hong Kong SAR Hong Kong Department of Health, 2000. As reported in the WPRO Country Profiles, 2000

Hungary Regular smoking measured by Central Statistical Office (KSH) and Dr L Pakozdi; information provided by Dr. E Podemaniczky, Head, Department of International Relations, National Institute of Oncology, 1998–99

Iceland Current tobacco smoking; World Health Organization Regional Office for Europe (2001). The European Tobacco Control Report: review of implementation of the Third Action Plan for a Tobacco Free Europe 1997–2001, Copenhagen

India SEAR Country Profiles, 2002

Indonesia SEAR Country Profiles, 2002

Iran Ministry of Health and Education, as reported in Eastern Mediterranean Tobacco Control Profile (survey 2002)

Iraq Current smoking; WHO (1997). Tobacco or health: a global status report. Geneva

Ireland Regular and occasional cigarette smoking measured by Survey of Lifestyle, Attitudes and Nutrition; Department of Health and Children/National University of Ireland. (1999). The National Health and Lifestyle Surveys. Dublin/Galway: Friel, S, et al.

Israel 11th World Conference on Tobacco OR Health: Abstracts Vol. 2 (Chicago, IL). 2000

Italy Regular daily cigarette smoking measured by ISTAT (Istituto Nazionale de Statistica); Italy's National Statistical Institute, April 2001

Jamaica Current smoking of cigars & cigarettes within 30 days before the interview; Wray, S R (1994). Prevalence and patterns of substance abusers: Neurobehavioural and social dimensions, Jamaica: The University of West Indies

Japan Current smoking of 100 cigarettes or more for the past six months measured by The National Livelihood Survey of 1998; Ministry of Health and Welfare (1999). National survey on smoking and health in Japan, 1999: Summary of findings. Tokyo

Jordan National Survey of Tobacco, MOH, 1999, as reported in Eastern Mediterranean Tobacco Control Profile (survey 2002)

Kazakhstan Current tobacco smoking; World Health Organization Regional Office for Europe (2001). The European Tobacco Control Report: review of implementation of the Third Action Plan for a Tobacco Free Europe 1997–2001, Copenhagen

Kenya Tobacco use in Nairobi; Wangai, P. (2000). Tobacco use in the city of Nairobi. *African Journal of Medical Practice*, 7(1), 13–20

Kiribati Hypertension and Diabetic Survey on South Tarawa and Betio, 1999, Dr Airam K.Metai, Director of Public Health Services and Kiribati National Focal Person for Tobacco or Health. As reported in the WPRO Country Profiles, 2000

Korea, Republic of Current smoking; Kim, I.S, et al. (2000). Trends of cigarette smoking of students, doctors and general population in Korea. 11th World Conference on Tobacco OR Health: Abstracts Vol. 2 (Chicago, IL)

Kuwait Family Health Survey, MOH, 1996, and Community Medicine Study, 2000, as reported in Eastern Mediterranean Tobacco Control Profile (survey 2002)

Kyrgyzstan Smoking in Bishkek measured by Dr. C. Bekbasarova (1998 is date of publication); WHO. (1998). Tobacco or health in Kyrgyzstan: Report of a WHO Mission to Bishkek

Lao, People's Dem. Rep. 1995 Pilot Study, Vientaine. As reported in the WPRO Country Profiles, 2000

Latvia Current tobacco smoking; World Health Organization Regional Office for Europe (2001). The European Tobacco Control Report: review of implementation of the Third Action Plan for a Tobacco Free Europe 1997–2001. Copenhagen

Lebanon National Survey of Smoking, 1998, as reported in Eastern Mediterranean Tobacco

Control Profile (survey 2002)

Lesotho Current cigarette smoking in rural areas; WHO (1997). Tobacco or health: a global status report. Geneva

Libyan Arab Jamahiriya Current smoking according to the Annual Report of the Center for Information and Documentation, General Secretary of Health and Social Welfare (1997)

Lithuania Current tobacco smoking; World Health Organization Regional Office for Europe (2001). The European Tobacco Control Report: review of implementation of the Third Action Plan for a Tobacco Free Europe 1997–2001, Copenhagen

Luxembourg Occasional and regular smoking measured by Fondation Luxembourgeoise Contre le Cancer and ILReS; information provided by Dr. Marie-Paul Prost-Heinisch of the Fondation Luxembourgeoise Contre le Cancer, 1998

Macedonia, FYR Current tobacco smoking; World Health Organization Regional Office for Europe (2001). The European Tobacco Control Report: review of implementation of the Third Action Plan for a Tobacco Free Europe 1997–2001, Copenhagen

Malawi Current smoking in a control group at the Queen Elizabeth Central Hospital in Blantyre, average age of 34 years (1996 is date of publication); Maher, D. et al. (1996). A survey of smoking in medical inpatients and controls in Blantyre, Malawi. Trop Doc, 26(3), 139

Malaysia Current smoking measured by the Second National Health and Morbidity Survey (NHMS2); information provided by Dr. Zarihah Zain, Ministry of Health, Penang State Health Department, 1996

Maldives SEAR Country Profiles, 2002

Malta Current smoking measured by the 1995 Population Census; information provided by Mr. Robert Mizzi, Central Office of Statistics

Mauritius *British Medical Journal*, 231, 345–349 (2000)

Mexico Current smoking for at least one month in urban areas, measured by the Instituto Nacional de Geografia, Estadistica e Informatica (INEGI); Secretaria de Salud, Direccion General de Epidemiologia. (1998). 1998 National Addictions Survey. Mexico: P K Morales

Mongolia ADRA & MOH Survey report, 2001

Morocco National Survey on Risk Factors for Cardiovascular Diseases, 2000, as reported in Eastern Mediterranean Tobacco Control Profile (survey 2002)

Mozambique

Myanmar 2001 Prevalence Study Draft Report, as reported in SEAR Country Profiles, 2002

Namibia Estimated tobacco use according to the Ministry of Health; WHO (1997). Tobacco or Health: a global status report, Geneva

Nauru Regular smoking (at least one cigarette per day) in rural and urban study areas; Li, N et al. (1994). Prevalence of coronary heart disease indicated by electrocardiogram abnormalities and risk factors in developing countries. *J Clin Epidemiol*, 47(6), 599–611

Nepal A study on Tobacco Economics in Nepal, Nepal Health Economics Association, WHO SEARO 2001, as reported in SEAR Country Profiles, 2002

Netherlands Current tobacco smoking; World Health Organization Regional Office for Europe (2001). The European Tobacco Control Report: review of implementation of the Third Action Plan for a Tobacco Free Europe 1997–2001, Copenhagen

New Zealand New Zealand Ministry of Health, 2001

Nigeria Cigarette smoking measured by a National Survey (1998 is date of publication); information provided by the Federal Ministry of Health

Niue 1980 Survey on smoking prevalence, as reported in the WPRO Country Profiles, 2000

Norway Current tobacco smoking; World Health Organization Regional Office for Europe (2001). The European Tobacco Control Report: review of implementation of the Third Action Plan for a Tobacco Free Europe 1997–2001, Copenhagen

Oman Gulf Family Health Survey, 1995, as reported in Eastern Mediterranean Tobacco Control Profile (survey 2002)

Pakistan National Health Survey, 1996, as reported in Eastern Mediterranean Tobacco Control Profile (survey 2002)

Palau Cigarette smoking; Palau Ministry of Health (1998). Palau Substance Abuse Needs Assessment (SANA). Palau: A Futterman

Panama Current smoking; WHO Pan American Health Organization Secretariat Report (1998). State of Tobacco Control in Latin America 1998

Papua New Guinea 1990 National Prevalence Survey, as reported in the WPRO Country Profiles, 2000

Paraguay Current smoking measured by a national survey of the Instituto de Investigaciones en Ciencias de la Salud; WHO Pan American Health Organization. (1992). Tobacco or Health: Status in the Americas. Washington, DC.

Peru Current smoking among the urban population; Rojas, M. <rojasmar@paho.org> (2000, June 19). Re: Smoking prevalence in Latin America. [data transfer via email].

Philippines 1999 National Nutrition Survey, as reported in the WPRO Country Profiles, 2000.

Poland Current tobacco smoking; World Health Organization Regional Office for Europe. (2001). The European Tobacco Control Report: review of implementation of the Third Action Plan for a Tobacco Free Europe 1997–2001, Copenhagen

Portugal Regular daily smoking, National Health Survey conducted by the Ministry of Health; Tobacco consumption, percent of population daily smokers. (1999), OECD Health Data 1999: A Comparative Analysis of 29 Countries. [CD-ROM], OECD

Puerto Rico Current smoking; Behavioral Risk Factor Surveillance System, Centers for Disease Control and Prevention (1999). 1998 Summary Prevalence Report, Atlanta, GA

Qatar Hamad Medical Center Survey, 1999, as reported in Eastern Mediterranean Tobacco Control Profile (survey 2002).

Republic of Moldova Current tobacco smoking; World Health Organization Regional Office for Europe (2001). The European Tobacco Control Report: review of implementation of the Third Action Plan for a Tobacco Free Europe 1997–2001, Copenhagen

Romania Current tobacco smoking; World Health Organization Regional Office for Europe (2001). The European Tobacco Control Report: review of implementation of the Third

Action Plan for a Tobacco Free Europe 1997–2001, Copenhagen.

Russian Federation Shalnova, S A, et al. Prevalence of smoking in Russia. Results of a survey of a nationally representative population sample, 1998

Rwanda Currently smoking 5 or more cigarettes per day, two main hospitals of Butare; Newton, R et al. (1996). Cancer in Rwanda. *Int J Cancer*, 66, 75–81

Saint Vincent and the Grenadines Current smoking, measured by the Ministry of Health's Risk Factor Survey; WHO Pan American Health Organization. (1997). Report: Risk factor survey in St. Vincent

Samoa 1994 Study on Urban Youth by UNDP and Statistics Department, as reported in the WPRO Country Profiles, 2000

San Marino Current smoking in the early 1990's; WHO. (1997). Tobacco or health: a global status report, Geneva

Sao Tome and Principe Smoking at least one cigarette per day (1998 is date of publication); Organizacao Mundial da Saude (1998). Analise da Situacao do Tabagismo em S. Tome E Principe, S. Tome

Saudi Arabia Family Health Survey, 1996, as reported in Eastern Mediterranean Tobacco Control Profile (survey 2002)

Senegal Tobacco and cigarette smoking in the District of Thiadiaye, Rural Senegal (1998 is date of publication); Kane, A et al. (1998). [Survey of smoking in the rural area of Thiadiaye, Senegal [French]. *Dakar Med.*, 43(1), 101–103.

Seychelles Current smoking of at least one cigarette per day; Bovet, P et al. (1997). The Seychelles Heart Study II: methods and basic findings. *Seychelles Medical & Dental Journal*, 5(1), 8–24

Sierra Leone Cigarette smoking, rural/agricultural communities of Njala Komboya and Kychum (1998 is date of publication); Williams, D E M, & Lisk, D R (1998). A high prevalence of hypertension in rural Sierra Leone. *WAJM*, 17(2), 85–90.

Singapore Daily smoking; Epidemiology and Disease Control Dept., Ministry of Health (1999). National Health Survey 1998, Singapore

Slovakia Smoking at least one cigarette a day or seven in a week; Urban, S et al. (1996). Epidemiology of smoking in Slovakia. Bratislava: Comenius University.

Slovenia Current smoking; Tos, N (forthcoming). Public Opinion Survey. Ljubljana: University of Ljubljana, 1999

Solomon Islands National Nutrition Survey, 1989, as reported in the WPRO Country Profiles, 2000

South Africa Daily and occasional smoking; Department of Health. (1998). South African Demographic and Health Survey: Preliminary Report. South Africa, A Ntsaluba

Spain Daily smoking in a nationally representative survey measured by the Ministry of Health; information provided by Dolors Marin, Ministerio de Sanidad y Consumo, Direccion General de Salud Publica, Subdireccion General de Epidemiologia, Promocion y Educacion para la Salud (Madrid)

Sri Lanka SEAR Country Profiles, 2002

Sudan 11th World Conference on Tobacco OR Health: Abstracts Vol. 2 (Chicago, IL). 2000

Swaziland Current smoking among parents of Form 1–5 students in four rural and urban regions; Pritchard, D (1999). Tobacco consumption among Swaziland high-school students and their parents and teachers. *SAMJ*, 89(5), 558–559.

Sweden Current tobacco smoking; World Health Organization Regional Office for Europe (2001). The European Tobacco Control Report: review of implementation of the Third Action Plan for a Tobacco Free Europe 1997–2001, Copenhagen

Switzerland Current tobacco smoking; World Health Organization Regional Office for Europe (2001). The European Tobacco Control Report: review of implementation of the Third Action Plan for a Tobacco Free Europe 1997–2001, Copenhagen

Syrian Arab Republic National Tobacco Survey, MOH, 1999, as reported in Eastern Mediterranean Tobacco Control Profile (survey 2002)

Thailand SEAR Country Profiles, 2002

Tonga Current smoking or smoking in the three months prior to the survey in almost all of Tonga; Woodward, A et al. (1994). Smoking in the Kingdom of Tonga: report from a national survey, *Tobacco Control*, 3, 41–45

Trinidad and Tobago Smoking at the time of survey; Miller, G J et al. (1989). Ethnicity and other characteristics predictive of coronary heart disease in a developing community: principal results of the St. James Survey, Trinidad. *Int J Epidemiol* 18(4), 808–817

Tunisia National Tobacco Survey, MOH, 1997, as reported in Eastern Mediterranean Tobacco Control Profile (survey 2002)

Turkey Current smoking; information provided by Prof. Nazmi Bilir, Hacettepe University Faculty of Medicine (sponsored by IDRC-Canada). 1996–99

Turkmenistan Regular daily smoking; Piha, T et al. (1993). Tobacco or health. World Health Stat Q, 46(3), 188–194

Tuvalu Current smoking; information provided by Dr. Harley Stanton; Tuomilehto, J et al. (1986). Smoking rates in the Pacific Islands. Bulletin of WHO, 64, 447–456

Uganda Smoking in a few suburbs of Kampala (1995 is date of data compilation), information provided by Dr. F Musoke; Wabinga, H R et al. (1995). Tobacco Smoking in Uganda, Markerere University Medical School.

Ukraine Institute of Cardiology, Ukrainian Academy of Medical Sciences, 1999

United Arab Emirates Family Health Survey, 1996, as reported in Eastern Mediterranean Tobacco Control Profile (survey 2002)

United Kingdom Current tobacco smoking; World Health Organization Regional Office for Europe (2001). The European Tobacco Control Report: review of implementation of the Third Action Plan for a Tobacco Free Europe 1997–2001, Copenhagen

United Rep. of Tanzania Consuming tobacco in three urban and rural regions; WHO Regional Office for Africa (1998). Tobacco in Tanzania: A situation analysis. Dar es Salaam: Dr. J Mbatia

United States of America Current cigarette smoking (having smoked 100+ cigarettes in lifetime and currently smoking every day or on some days); Centers for Disease Control and Prevention (2000). Cigarette smoking among adults - United States 1999. National Health Interview Survey.

Uruguay Current smoking measured by National Institute of Statistics (INE); Data provided during an interview with Dr. Helmut Kasdorf, President, Uruguayan Anti-Tobacco Association (4 May 1999)

Uzbekistan Current tobacco smoking; World Health Organization Regional Office for Europe (2001). The European Tobacco Control Report: review of implementation of the Third Action Plan for a Tobacco Free Europe 1997–2001, Copenhagen

Vanuatu 1998 National Noncommunicable Diseases Survey, as reported in the WPRO Country Profiles, 2000

Venezuela Daily and occasional smoking of 20 cigarettes or less; information provided by Natasha Herrera through the WHO Tobacco or Health Database.

Vietnam Vietnam Living Standards Study, General Statistics Office, 2002;S2, 62

Yemen Cigarette smoking (1997 is date of publication); Al-Motawakel, A. (1997). Smoking in Yemen. Sana'a: Al Thawra Modern General Hospital

Yugoslavia Current tobacco smoking; World Health Organization Regional Office for Europe. (2001). The European Tobacco Control Report: review of implementation of the Third Action Plan for a Tobacco Free Europe 1997–2001. Copenhagen.

Zambia Estimated tobacco smoking measured by Central Statistical Office; Ministry of Health. (1998). Tobacco and health situation in Zambia among adolescents and young adults: growing up without tobacco. Lusaka: S Makono

Zimbabwe Cigarette smoking; Watts, et al. (1997). Education, occupation and health status of people of age five years or more living in a high density urban area in Zimbabwe *Cent Afr J Med*, 43(9), 260–264

Corrao MA, Guidon GE, Sharma N, Shokoohi DF (eds), *Tobacco Control Country Profiles*, American Cancer Society, Atlanta, GA, USA, 2000

World Health Organization, *The European Report on Tobacco Control Policy*, EUR/01/5020906/8 February 2002

World Health Organization, *Country Profiles on Tobacco Control in the Eastern Mediterranean Region*, EMRO, May 2002

CLIPBOARD QUOTE

Ibison D, Rothmans' joint deal opens heavenly gates, *Window*, Hong Kong, 16 Oct 1992:4

SMOKING TRENDS

Japan: *Japan Tobacco Annual Reports*

Japan: (the late) Hirayama T, personal communication, 1995

UK: Tobacco Advisory Council. In Wald N, Nicolaides-Bouman A. *UK Smoking Statistics*. Second edition, 1991

UK: *Living in Britain*, General Household Surveys, 1980–1998

USA: US Department of Health and Human Services, *National Health Interview Survey. In Women and Smoking: A Report of the Surgeon General*, US Department of Health and Human Services, Centers for Disease Control and Prevention, National Center for Chronic Disease Prevention and Health Promotion, Office on Smoking and Health, 2001

USA: *Morbidity and Mortality Weekly Report*, Cigarette smoking among adults–United States, 1999, Vol 50 (40): 869–73, October 12, 2001

PHYSICIANS WHO SMOKE

Corrao MA, Guidon GE, Sharma N, Shokoohi DF (eds) *Tobacco Control Country Profiles*, American Cancer Society, Atlanta, GA, USA, 2000

Czech: Sovinova H, *Treatment of tobacco dependence in the Czech Republic*. Public and private sector partnerships to reduce tobacco dependence. Prague, Czech Republic, 13–14 December 2001

Japan: Ohida T, Sakurai H, Mochizuki Y, Kamal AMM, Takemura S, Minowa M, Kawahara K, *Smoking Prevalence and Attitudes Toward Smoking Among Japanese Physicians* JAMA. 2001;285:2643–2648

UK: British Medical Association, *Smoking prevalence of British doctors*, 1999

TEXT

Scull R, Bright Future Predicted for Asia Pacific. *World Tobacco*, Sept 1986:35

4 Female Smoking

MAIN MAP

Sources as for Map 3 MALE SMOKING

CLIPBOARD

Thornton RE, The smoking behaviour of women, BAT (File B3183) 105501517
- 565. Study of motivational differences between men and women smokers.
12 Nov 1976, research report (RD 1410)

5 Youth

MAPS

The Global Youth Tobacco Survey Collaborative Group, *Tobacco Use Among
Youth: A cross country comparison*, Tobacco Control, in press

Wick Warren, Centers for Disease Control and Prevention, Atlanta, USA
(personal communication), 2002

40% OF CHILDREN...

Calculation by Dr Alan Lopez, WHO, for WHO Consultation on
Environmental Tobacco Smoke (ETS) and Child Health, Geneva, 11–14
January 1999

CLIPBOARD

Johnston ME, Philip Morris (PM) Bates No. 1000390803. *Young Smokers
Prevalence Trends, Implications and Related Demographic Trends*, 31 March 1981

6 Cigarette Consumption

MAIN MAP

Per capita cigarette consumption figures constructed from production, trade
(import and export) and population data.

Data sources include:

ERC Statistics International plc, *The World Cigarette Market: The 1998 Survey*,
Suffolk, Great Britain, 1999

ECOWAS Social and Economic Indicators 1998, Economic Community of West
African States, 1999

Food and Agriculture Organization of the United Nations (FAO), FaoStat
Statistical databases. http://apps.fao.org/

Interstate Statistical Committee of the Commonwealth of Independent States.
Official Statistics of the Countries of the Commonwealth of Independent States, CD-
ROM, 2000-5 http://www.unece.org/stats/cisstat/cd-offst.htm

United Nations dataset *World Population Prospects 1950–2050* (2000 revision),
New York, United Nations Population Division, 2000

United Nations Industrial Commodity Production Statistics Database,
1950–1998, CD-ROM, prepared by the Industrial Statistics Section,
Statistics Division, 2000, New York, USA

United Nations Statistics Division. Commodity Trade Statistics Data Base
(COMTRADE) http://esa.un.org/unsd/pubs/

United States Department of Agriculture, Economic Research Service, *Tobacco
Statistics* (94012), April 1994 and June 1996
http://usda.mannlib.cornell.edu/data-sets/specialty/94012/

United States Department of Agriculture, Foreign Agricultural Service, *Tobacco:
World Markets and Trade,* various issues
http://www.fas.usda.gov/currwmt.html

United States Department of Agriculture, Foreign Agricultural Service. *Attaché
Reports,* various issues
http://www.fas.usda.gov/scriptsw/attacherep/default.asp

United States Department of Agriculture, World Cigarette Consumption,
selected countries, 1960–95, Tobacco Statistics Stock #94012 Economic
Research Service, Table 170, 1996

GLOBAL CIGARETTE CONSUMPTION

Proctor RN, personal communication, 2001

McGinn AP, The Nicotine Cartel, *World Watch* Vol. 10, No 4; 1997:18–27

RISING NUMBERS

Smoking and Health in China,*1996 National Prevalence Survey of Smoking Pattern*,
China Science and Technology Press, Beijing, China, 1996:10

Peto R, Monitoring the Large Increase in Tobacco Deaths, 6th National
Symposium on Smoking and Health. Guangzhou, China, 3–5 November 1995

TOP 5 COUNTRIES

ERC, *The World Cigarette Market: The 1999 Survey*, ERC Group plc, 2000

TEXT

Economic Research Service, Cigarette consumption continues to slip,
Agricultural Outlook, January–February, 2001

ERC, *The World Cigarette Market: The 1999 Survey*, ERC Group plc, 2000

7 Health Risks

MAIN GRAPHIC

British Medical Bulletin; Vol 52, No 1, 1996. Published for the British Council by
the Royal Society of Medicine Press Limited. Scientific Editors: Sir Richard
Doll and Sir John Crofton

Doll R, Peto R, Wheatley K, Gray R, Sutherland I. Mortality in relation to
smoking: 40 years' observation on male British doctors, *British Medical
Journal*, 1994; 309:901–11

American Cancer Society (CPSII) in Surgeon General's Report. *Reducing the
Health Consequences of Smoking: 25 Years of Progress*, US Dept of Health and
Human Services, 1989. Publication No CDC 89-8411

GASP! Inside Story, Comic Company, 1997

BABES IN THE WOMB

Ernster V, Kaufman K, Nichter M, Samet J, Yoon SY. Women and Tobacco:
Moving from policy to action, *Bulletin of the World Health Organization*, 2000,
78 (7) 891-901

DEADLY CHEMICALS

Tobacco Ingredients in All Brands, Philip Morris. 11 Jan 2001

Crawford MA, Balch GI, Mermelstein R and The Tobacco Control Network
Writing Group, *Responses to tobacco control policies among youth*, Tobacco
Control 2002;11:14-19

CLIPBOARD

Private statement: Mellman AJ, 1983. In: *Tobacco Industry Quotes On Nicotine And
Addiction From Recently Released Documents*, Campaign for Tobacco-Free Kids,
Oct 26, 1999

Sworn testimony: 7 CEOs of American Tobacco, Brown & Williamson Tobacco
Company, Liggett Group, Lorillard Tobacco Company, Philip Morris, RJR
Tobacco Company, US Tobacco Company, to House Commerce Committee,
USA, 14 April 1994

8 Passive Smoking

MAIN GRAPHIC

National Cancer Institute, Health effects of exposure to Environmental Tobacco
Smoke: The Report of the California Environmental Protection Agency,
Smoking and Tobacco Control Monograph no. 10. Bethesda, MD. U.S.
Department of Health and Human Services, National Institutes of Health,
National Cancer Institute. NIH Pub. No. 99-4645, 1999

*World Health Organization International Consultation on Environmental Tobacco Smoke
(ETS) and Child Health*, 11–14 January 1999, World Health Organization,
Tobacco Free Initiative Consultation Report, Geneva, Switzerland.
WHO/NCD/TFI/99.10: 6-11

CHILDREN EXPOSED TO PASSIVE SMOKING AT HOME
The Global Youth Tobacco Survey Collaborative Group, *Tobacco Use among Youth: A cross country comparison*, Tobacco Control, in press

NUMBERS AFFECTED BY PASSIVE SMOKING
National Cancer Institute. Health effects of exposure to Environmental Tobacco Smoke: The Report of the California Environmental Protection Agency. *Smoking and Tobacco Control Monograph no. 10.* Bethesda, MD. U.S. Department of Health and Human Services, National Institutes of Health, National Cancer Institute. NIH Pub. No. 99–4645, 1999

CLIPBOARD
For internal use only: Philip Morris Issues Training Manual, 30 May–1 June 1995
Secret poll: [116] The Roper Organization, *A Study of Public Attitudes Towards Cigarette Smoking and the Tobacco Industry in 1978*, Vol. 1, 1978. In Glantz SA, Slade J, Bero LA, Hanauer P, Barnes DE (eds), *The Cigarette Papers*, University of California Press, 1996

TEXT
Doll R, Peto J, *Asbestos – Effects on health exposure to asbestos.* Her Majesty's Stationary Office, 1985
Physicians for a Smoke-Free Canada, *Questions and Answers on Health Effects of Second-hand Smoke*, April 2001
Smoke Free Workplaces: Improving the health and well-being of people at work. European Conference on Smoke-free Workplaces. Conference statement, 10–11 May 2001 Berlin, Germany
The Scoth Report: 1998 Report of the Scientific Committee on Tobacco and Health, Department of Health, UK 98/086
World Health Organization, *International Consultation on Environmental Tobacco Smoke (ETS) and Child Health*, 11–14 January 1999, WHO/TFI, Geneva, Switzerland, WHO/NCD/TFI//99.10
Action on Smoking and Health, UK, *Passive Smoking: A summary of the evidence*,October 2001, http://www.ash.org.uk/
Ong E, Glantz SA. Hirayama's work has stood the test of time. *Bulletin of the World Health Organization*, 2000, 78 (7): 938–9

9 Deaths

MAIN MAP, TOTAL DEATHS and PAST AND FUTURE
Ezzati M, Lopez A, Mortality and burden of disease attributable to smoking and oral tobacco use, Global and Regional estimates for 2000, to appear in *Comparative Risk Assessment*, World Health Organization, 2002

CLIPBOARD
Campbell Johnson ltd. A Public Relations Strategy, Bates No. 2501160781/0803, 20 Nov 1978
http://www.pmdocs.com/getallimg.asp?DOCID=2501160781/0803

TEXT
Peto R, Lopez AD. *Future Worldwide Health Effects of Current Smoking Patterns*, Chapter 18. In Eds Koop CE, Pearson CE, Schwarz MR. *Critical issues in global health,* Jossey-Bass, 2001:155

Part Two:
THE COSTS OF TOBACCO

10 Costs to the economy

MAIN MAP
Australia: Australian Medical Association. In: AMA says tobacco is putting pressure on public hospitals, Australian Broadcasting Corporation, 22 July 1999
Canada: Kaiserman MJ, *Chronic Diseases in Canada. The Cost of Smoking in Canada*, 1991, Health Protection Branch - Laboratory Centre for Disease Control, Canada, 1997, Vol 18, no 1
http://www.hcsc.gc.ca/hpb/lcdc/publicat/cdic/cdic181/cd181c_e.html
Downloaded 30 December 2001
China: Jin SG, Lu BY, Yan DY, Fu ZY, Jiang Y, Li W. An evaluation on smoking-induced health costs in China (1988–1989), *Biomedical and Environmental Sciences*, 1995, 8, 342–349
Germany: Ruff LK, Volmer T, Nowak D, Meyer A, The economic impact of smoking in Germany. *European Respiratory Journal*, 2000 Sep;16(3):385–90
UK: ASH UK, *Smoking and Economics, Basic Facts No. 3*, downloaded 30 December 2001, http://www.ash.org.uk/
USA: Centers for Disease Control and Prevention, USA, Annual Smoking-Attributable Mortality, Years of Potential Life Lost, and Economic Costs, United States, 1995–1999, *Morbidity and Mortality Weekly Report*, 12 April 2002, 51(14):300–303

COSTS OF FIRES CAUSED BY SMOKING
Leistikow BN, Martin DC, Milano CE, Fire injuries, disasters, and costs from cigarettes and cigarette lights: A global overview, *Preventive Medicine*, 2000, 31:~91

EVERY YEAR, 1,000,000 FIRES …
Leistikow BN, Martin DC, Milano CE. Fire injuries, disasters, and costs from cigarettes and cigarette lights: A global overview. *Preventive Medicine*, 2000, 31:~91

TRASH COLLECTED IN THE USA
Center for Marine Conservation. In: Shoreline Cleanup Yielded 4 Million Pieces Of Trash. *Detroit Free Press*, 21 June 1996 Section: NWS:4A.

CHINA 1987: THE WORST FOREST FIRE IN THE WORLD CAUSED BY CIGARETTES
Reuter, Sacked foreign minister was in the hospital during the blaze, *South China Morning Post*, 8 June 1987
Associated Press, Eleven face court after death fires, *South China Morning Post*, 14 June 1988:8

WORKPLACE SMOKING COSTS THE USA US$47 BILLION EVERY YEAR.
Office of Technology Assessment, *Smoking-related deaths and financial costs: estimates for 1990*, revised ed. Washington DC: Office of Technology Assessment, 1993

AVERAGE DAYS OFF SICK PER YEAR
Halpern MT, Shikiar R, Rentz AM, Khan ZM. Impact of smoking status on workplace absenteeism and productivity, *Tobacco Control* 2001;10:233–238 (Autumn)

CLIPBOARDS
REFLECTING 5.23 YEARS...
Public Finance: Balance of Smoking in the Czech Republic, report
    commissioned by Philip Morris,Czech Republic, 2001
PHILIP MORRIS APOLOGIZES...
Fairclough G, *The Wall Street Journal*, 26 July 2001

ANNUAL COST OF LOSS OF TIME OFF WORK
Medical Journal of Australia, 1994;161:407–1. Reported in Minerva, *British
    Medical Journal*, 22 Oct 1994: 6961, vol 309:1098

SMOKING ACCOUNTED FOR OVER 6–7% OF TOTAL HEALTH CARE
    COSTS IN THE USA IN 1999
Warner KE, Hodgson TA, Carroll CE. Medical costs of smoking in the United
    States: estimates, their validity, and their implications, *Tobacco Control 1999*;
    8:290–300 (Autumn).
Miller VP, Ernst C, Collin F, Smoking-attributable medical care costs in the
    USA, *Social Science and Medicine* 1999;48:375–91.
Max W. The financial impact of smoking on health-related costs: a review of the
    literature. *American Journal of Health Promotion* 2001;15:321–31
Centers for Disease Control and Prevention, USA, Annual Smoking-
    Attributable Mortality, Years of Potential Life Lost, and Economic Costs,
    United States, 1995–1999, *Morbidity and Mortality Weekly Report*, 12 April
    2002, 51(14):300–303

11 Costs to the Smoker

MAIN MAP
Guindon GE, S Tobin S, Yach D, Trends and affordability of cigarette prices:
    ample room for tax increases and related health gains. *Tobacco Control
    2002*;11:35–43. Data from Economist Intelligence Unit; calculations made by
    World Health Organization.
Corrao MA, Guindon GE, Cokkinides V, Sharma N, Building the evidence base
    for global tobacco control, *Bulletin of the World Health Organization*, 2000, 78
    (7). Special Theme – Tobacco
Joossens L, Prices and tax incidence of a pack of 20 of the most popular price
    category in the EU in US$ on January 1, 1998. Data from European
    Commission.
Sweanor D, Global cigarette taxes and prices. Average Retail Cigarette Price
    and Total Taxes per Pack, Selected Countries, December 31, 1996. *Smoking
    and Health Action Foundation*, April 30, 1997
White A. A pack of Marlboro costs..., Partnership Programme, Essential
    Action's Taking on Tobacco campaign. Survey, 14 countries, Dec 2000.
    <awhite@essential.org>

A HARD DAY'S SMOKE
Guindon GE, S Tobin S, Yach D. Trends and affordability of cigarette prices:
    ample room for tax increases and related health gains. *Tobacco Control
    2002*;11:35–43

A PACK OF MARLBORO OR EQUIVALENT ...
White A. A pack of Marlboro costs... Partnership Programme, Essential
    Action's Taking on Tobacco campaign. Survey, 14 countries, Dec 2000.
    <awhite@essential.org>

MINHANG, CHINA
Gong LY, Koplan JP, Feng W, Chen CH, Zheng P, Harris JR, Cigarette smoking
    in China. *Journal of the American Medical Association* 1995; 274:1232–4

TEXT
Shanghai: Anon, Expenditure on cigarettes, *Oriental Daily News* 5 May 1990:20

Part Three:
THE TOBACCO TRADE

12 Growing Tobacco

MAIN MAP
Food and Agriculture Organization, Tobacco Leaves, Area Harvested
    (Hectares), 2001, FAOSTAT Database Results, FAO website accessed
    January 2002, http://apps.fao.org/lim500/nph-
    wrap.pl?Production.Crops.Primary&Domain=SUA
SYMBOL
Corrao MA, Guidon GE, Sharma N, Shokoohi DF (eds) *Tobacco Control Country
    Profiles*, American Cancer Society, Atlanta, GA, USA, 2000

FIVE COUNTRIES
Food and Agriculture Organization, Tobacco Leaves, Area Harvested
    (Hectares), 2001. FAOSTAT Database Results, FAO website accessed
    January 2002, http://apps.fao.org/lim500/nph-
    wrap.pl?Production.Crops.Primary&Domain=SUA

DEFORESTATION
Geist H, Global assessment of reforestation related to tobacco farming, *Tobacco
    Control 1999*, 8:18–28

LEADING PRODUCERS OF TOBACCO LEAVES
Food and Agriculture Organization, Tobacco Leaves, Production (Metric Tons),
    2001, FAOSTAT Database Results, FAO website accessed January 2002,
    http://apps.fao.org/lim500/nph-
    wrap.pl?Production.Crops.Primary&Domain=SUA

TEXT
Corrao MA, Guidon GE, Sharma N, Shokoohi DF (eds), *Tobacco Control Country
    Profiles*. American Cancer Society, Atlanta, GA, USA, 2000
USDA, Tobacco and the Economy, AER–789, Economic Research Service,
    September 2000
USDA, Economic Research Service, Tobacco Statistics (94102) Table 156 ,
    World tobacco acreage, and Table 157, World tobacco production, selected
    countries, 1960–1995. USDA website accessed January 2002,
    http://www.ers.usda.gov/data/sdp/view.asp?f=specialty/94012/
Jha P and Chaloupka FJ , *Tobacco Control in Developing Countries*, Oxford
    University Press 2000, pp. 315–317
Global Leaf, *Barren Harvest: The Costs of Tobacco Farming*, Campaign for Tobacco
    Free Kids, USA 2001

13 Manufacturing Tobacco

MAIN MAP
United Nations Industrial Development Organisation (UNIDO), Statistics and
    Information Networks Branch, Industrial Statistics Database 2001, 3-digit
    level of ISIC Code, United Nations International Standard Industrial
    Classification (Revision 2) at the 3-digit level: 314 Tobacco, 2002
    http://www.unido.org/doc/50314.htmls

WHERE THE TOBACCO DOLLAR GOES, 1997
USDA, *Tobacco and the economy: Farms, jobs and communities*, Gale FH, Foreman L,
    and Capehart T: *Agricultural Report* Number 789, Economic Research Service,
    2000

LESS TOBACCO PER CIGARETTE

USDA, *Tobacco Situation and Outlook Report* (TBS 250, Table 28 – Estimated leaf used for cigarettes by kind of tobacco, 1960–2000 (total domestic farm-sales weight), September 2001

ADDITIVES

Philip Morris Web Page

http://www.pmusa.com/DisplayPageWithTopic.asp?ID=42

TEXT

USDA, Economic Research Service, Tobacco Statistics (94102) Table 156 , World tobacco acreage, and Table 167, World cigarette production, selected countries, 1960–1995. USDA website accessed January 2002, http://www.ers.usda.gov/data/sdp/view.asp?f=specialty/94012/

United Nations Industrial Development Organisation (UNIDO), Statistics and Information Networks Branch, Industrial Statistics Database 2001, 3-digit level of ISIC Code, United Nations International Standard Industrial Classification (Revision 2) at the 3-digit level: 314 Tobacco, 2002. http://www.unido.org/doc/50314.htmls

Buck D, Godfrey C, Raw M, and Sutton M, *Tobacco and Jobs: The impact of reducing consumption on employment in the UK*, May 1995

Gale FH, Foreman L, and Capehart T, Tobacco and the economy: Farms, jobs and communities, *Agricultural Report* Number 789, Economic Research Service, USDA 2000

14 Tobacco Companies

MAIN MAP

ERC. *The World Cigarette Market: The 1999 Survey*, ERC Group plc, 2000

DMG World Media (UK) Ltd, *World Tobacco File*, 4th Edition, 2000, Surrey, United Kingdom

Monopolies Privatisation: A Realm of Risks and Rewards, *Tobacco Journal International*, 11 August 2000

USDA, Foreign Agricultural Service. In: Monopolies still standing: monopolies in the Middle East and Africa, *Tobacco Journal Online*, 05/2000

Corrao MA, Guidon GE, Sharma N, Shokoohi DF (eds), *Tobacco Control Country Profiles*, American Cancer Society, Atlanta, GA, USA, 2000

THE BIG FIVE

ERC. *The World Cigarette Market: The 1999 Survey*, ERC Group plc, 2000

DMG World Media (UK) Ltd, *World Tobacco File*, 4th Edition, 2000, Surrey, UK

CLIPBOARD

The Times, London, 14 October 1994, in Hammond R, *Russia*, Center for Communications, Health & the Environment

TEXT

Monopolies Privatisation: A Realm of Risks and Rewards, *Tobacco Journal International*, 8 Nov 2000

Hammond R, Consolidation in the tobacco industry. Industry Watch, *Tobacco Control 1998*, 7:426–428

CNTC, Philip Morris Sign Agreement of Intent on Cooperation, STMA Information Center. *Tobacco China*, 7 February 2002

Chaloupka FJ, Laixuthai A, US Trade Policy and Cigarette Smoking in Asia, National Bureau of Economic Research, June 1996. Working paper number 5,543

Havrylyshyn O, and McGettigan D, 1998 *Privatization in transition countries: Lessons of the first decade*, IMF Working Paper WP/99/6, Washington DC, World Bank Publication Series.

Nellis J, 1998 Privatization in transition economies: An update, pp13–22 in *Case by case privatization in the Russian Federation: Lessons from international experience*, World Bank discussion paper No. 385, edited by H.G. Broadman, Washington DC World Bank: 13–22

Kikeri S, 1998, *Privatization and labor: What happens to workers when governments divest?*, World Bank Technical Paper No.396

15 Tobacco Trade

MAIN MAP

United States Department of Agriculture, Foreign Agricultural Service, *Tobacco: World Markets and Trade*, various issues http://www.fas.usda.gov/currwmt.html

United Nations Statistics Division. Commodity Trade Statistics Data Base (COMTRADE), http://esa.un.org/unsd/pubs/

TOP 10 CIGARETTE IMPORTING COUNTRIES

United Nations Statistics Division. Commodity Trade Statistics Data Base (COMTRADE) http://esa.un.org/unsd/pubs/

TOP 10 LEAF EXPORTERS/IMPORTERS

Food and Agriculture Organization of the United Nations (FAO). FaoStat Statistical databases. http://apps.fao.org/ [FAOSTAT code 0826]

US IMPORTS AND EXPORTS: TOBACCO LEAVES

United Nations Statistics Division. Commodity Trade Statistics Data Base (COMTRADE) http://esa.un.org/unsd/pubs/

Food and Agriculture Organization,United Nations (FAO), FaoStat Statistical databases, http://apps.fao.org/

US IMPORTS AND EXPORTS: CIGARETTES

United Nations Statistics Division. Commodity Trade Statistics Data Base (COMTRADE) http://esa.un.org/unsd/pubs/

TEXT

Food and Agriculture Organization of the United Nations (FAO). FaoStat Statistical databases, http://apps.fao.org/

China: Ni Y, National Tobacco Conference, Beijing, China. Reported in *Tobacco China*, 1 February 2001

16 Smuggling

MAIN MAP

Jha P and Chaloupka FJ, *Tobacco control in developing countries*, Table 15.3 Estimates of price, smuggling and transparency, Oxford University Press, 2000:373

ROUTES

Illegal pathways to illegal profits. The Big Cigarette Companies and International Smuggling, Campaign for Tobacco Free Kids. http://tobaccofreekids.org/campaign/global/framework/docs/Smuggling.pdf, downloaded 14 February 2002

Personal communication with Luk Joossens and Eric LeGresley, 2002

TACKLING TOBACCO SMUGGLING

Tackling Tobacco Smuggling, HM Customs and Excise, HM Treasury, UK, March 2000

LOST REVENUE

Commission of Enquiry into the community transit system. Brussels European Parliament, 1997 (4 volumes), in Joossens L and Raw M, Cigarette smuggling in Europe: who really benefits? *Tobacco Control 1998*,7:66–71, Spring

GLOBAL SMUGGLING

Joossens L. *How to combat tobacco smuggling through the WHO Framework Convention on Tobacco Control*, presentation at the Second World Conference on Modern Criminal Investigation, Organized Crime and Human Rights, Durban, South Africa, 7 December 2001

CHINA

Korski T. Tax cuts to curb cigarette smuggling, *South China Morning Post* (Business Post), 5 May 1997:1, in Mackay J. Smoking in China: "the limits of space", [editorial] *Tobacco Control*, Summer 1997; Vol 6, No 2:77–79

CLIPBOARD

BAT doc. 302000021, 1989, in *Illegal pathways to illegal profits. The Big Cigarette Companies and International Smuggling*, Campaign for Tobacco Free Kids:4, http://tobaccofreekids.org/campaign/global/framework/docs/Smuggling.pdf

TEXT

Joossens L, *Technical Paper on Tobacco and Smuggling - Questions and Answers*, WHO, Geneva, 1998
Boucher P. Rendez-vous 129. Rendez-vous with Luk Joossens. Consultant about tobacco smuggling for WHO and UICC, Brussels, Belgium. 19 February 2002.
Illegal pathways to illegal profits. The Big Cigarette Companies and International Smuggling, Campaign for Tobacco Free Kids. http://tobaccofreekids.org/campaign/global/framework/docs/Smuggling.pdf, downloaded 14 February 2002
World Bank Report, *Curbing the epidemic. Economics of tobacco control*, Washington DC, June 1999
Joossens L, Raw M. Cigarette smuggling in Europe: who really benefits? *Tobacco control 1998*, 7:66–71

Part Four: PROMOTION

17 Tobacco Industry Promotion

MAIN MAP

ERC. *The World Cigarette Market: The 1999 Survey*, ERC Group Plc, 2000
DMG World Media (UK) Ltd, *World Tobacco File*, 4th Edition, ISBN: 1-84313-006-8, 2000, Surrey, UK
The Maxwell Report, *1999 International Tobacco Report*, Part One (28 April 2000) and Part Two (28 July 2000), John C. Maxwell, Jr., 4703 Rolfe Road Richmond, VA, 23226, USA

HOW THE ADVERTISING DOLLAR IS SPENT IN THE USA

US Federal Trade Commission Cigarette Report for 2000, Washington DC, USA, 2002

CHANGES IN CIGARETTE MARKETING EXPENDITURE

US Federal Trade Commission Cigarette Report for 2000, Washington DC, USA, 2002

WORLD'S MOST POPULAR BRANDS

DMG World Media (UK) Ltd, *World Tobacco File*, 4th Edition, ISBN: 1-84313-006-8, 2000, Surrey, UK

CLIPBOARD

Whitbread M, Sponsorship Manager, Gallaher International (re: Silk Cut South China Sea Race), *South China Morning Post*, Hong Kong. 22 February 1986

20TH CENTURY

AdAge.Com http://www.adage.com/news.cms?newsid=33975

TEXT

How Do You Sell Death? Campaign for Tobacco Free Kids, Washington, DC, 2001

18 Internet Sales

WHERE ARE THE GOODS?

ASH UK, Cigarettes on the Internet: A Survey by Action on Smoking and Health (ASH), Published 13 June 2001, http://www.ash.org.uk/

INTERNET CIGARETTE SEARCH

Mackay J, Google, 27 March 2002

INTERNET CIGARETTE VENDORS

Ribisl KM, Kim AE, Williams RS, Web sites selling cigarettes: how many are there in the USA and what are their sales practices? *Tobacco Control 2001*, 10:352–359 (Winter)
Kim AE, Ribisl KM, Hoffman RS, *Sales practices of Internet cigarette vendors: Are they adequate to prevent minors from buying cigarettes online?*, The 128th Annual Meeting of APHA, November 2000
Kurt M. Ribisl, Annice E. Kim, and Rebecca S. Williams. Are the Sales Practices of Internet Cigarette Vendors Good Enough to Prevent Sales to Minors? *American Journal of Public Health* 2002 92: 940–941

CLIPBOARD

Tobacco giant under scrutiny for website, *Australian Associated Press*, 12 December 2000

HK CUSTOMS AND EXCISE QUOTE

ASH UK, *Buying cigarettes on the Internet: A survey by Action on Smoking and Health* (ASH), 13 June 2001, http://www.ash.org.uk/

WOW!!!!!!!!!!!!!!!

http://www.discount-cigarettes.org/consumers.html, downloaded 27 March 2002

TEXT

Streitfeld D, Online Tobacco Sales Ignite Fight Over Taxes, *The Washington Post*, Page A01, 29 August 2000
Connolly GN, editorial: Smokes and cyberspace: a public health disaster in the making. *Tobacco Control 2001*, 10:299, Winter

19 Politics

CLIPBOARDS ON MAP
SMALL SHOPKEEPERS...
Philip Morris 10 August 1990. Industry response to, and impact of, anti-tobacco legislation in Canada, *Landman Collection*, landman/2026230531-0540.
WE HAVE GOT THE UNIONS...
Philip Morris: The Perspective of PM International on Smoking and Health Issues, 27 March 1985, *Landman Collection* landman/2023268351-8364: 7
PHILIP MORRIS AND THE INDUSTRY...
Philip Morris Corporate Affairs Plan. 25 November 1987, *Landman Collection* landman/2501254715-4723

TURNING NOW…
Philip Morris: The Perspective of PM International on Smoking and Health
  Issues, 27 March 1985, *Landman Collection* landman/2023268351-8364
THE INTERNATIONAL TOBACCO GROWERS…
INFOTAB, 1988, Bloxcidge J, fax to INFOTAB Board Members, 11 October
  1988, British American Tobacco Company 502555415-5417, Guildford
  Document Depository

QUOTES
UNLESS COUNTERVAILING STEPS…
RJ Reynolds document, 1978, *Landman Collection*, Bates No. 500851221-
  500851262.
WHAT ARE WE TRYING TO ACCOMPLISH?
Document Type: Report, Date: 03/20/1990, Author: N/A, Title: Top Secret
  Operation Rainmaker, Site: Philip Morris document site, Bates No.
  2048302227/2230
  http://www.pmdocs.com/getallimg.asp?DOCID=2048302227/2230

BUYING INFLUENCE
Watch, Public Citizen, USA, 1998
  http://www.citizen.org/congress/civjus/prod_liability/tobacco/articles.cfm
  ?ID=908

BUYING FAVOURS
Common Cause: Buying Influence, Selling Death, 14 March 2001

TEXT
Common Cause: Buying Influence, Selling Death, 14 March 2001
Neuman M, Bitton A, Glantz S. Tobacco industry strategies for influencing
  European Community tobacco advertising legislation, *The Lancet* 2002, 359:
  1323–30
  http://www.thelancet.com/journal/vol359/iss9314/full/llan.359.9314.edit
  orial_and_review.20721.1

20 Smokers' Rights Organisations

MAIN MAP
TOBACCOpedia: The Online Tobacco Encyclopedia, Search 21 February 2002,
  http://158.232.12.95/cgi-
  bin/search/seek.cgi?search=CAT&Category=Tobacco%20industry%20%26
  %20supporters%3AAssociations%2C%20organizations
Mackay J, search 21 February 2002, http://158.232.12.95/cgi-
  bin/search/seek.cgi?search=CAT&Category=Tobacco%20industry%20%26
  %20supporters%3AAssociations%2C%20organizations
ASH UK. *Fact Sheet No. 18: The Tobacco Industry*, http://www.ash.org.uk/
  February 2002

CLIPBOARDS
TO SUM UP…
Philip Morris: The Perspective of PM International on Smoking and Health
  Issues, 27 March 1985, quoted in *Landman Collection* landman/2023268351-
  8364, page 8
FIRST WE MUST…
Philip Morris: The Perspective of PM International on Smoking and Health
  Issues, 27 march 1985, quoted in *Landman Collection* landman/2023268351-
  8634
WE TRY TO KEEP PHILIP MORRIS OUT OF THE MEDIA…
Walls T. Philip Morris. Grasstops Government Relations, 30 March 1993. Bates
  No. 2024023252/3265,
  http://www.pmdocs.com/getallimg.asp?DOCID=2024023252/3265

SMOKERS ARE NOT…
RJ Reynolds document 22 December 1978. Bates No. 500851221-500851262
IN AUSTRALIA TOO
Philip Morris: The Perspective of PM International on Smoking and Health
  Issues, 27 March 1985, quoted in *Landman Collection* landman/2023268351-
  8364

TEXT
Philip Morris document 13 December, 1988. From *Landman Collection* :
  2021596422-2021596432: 7
Landman A, 26 March 2002, Comments pertaining to Bates No. 2045741537-
  1539

21 Tobacco Industry Documents

MAIN MAP
Authors search using country names, Legacy Foundation site, April 2002,
  http://legacy.library.ucsf.edu/

CLIPBOARDS
OUR WORK IN SENEGAL…
Whist A. Philip Morris Memorandum. 17 December 1986. Bates No.
  2025431401/1406
  http://www.pmdocs.com/getallimg.asp?DOCID=2025431401/1406
WORK TO DEVELOP…
Philip Morris, 1987, as quoted in *Voices of Truth*, Volume 2
A LAW PROHIBITING…
Whist A., Philip Morris Memorandum. 17 December 1986, Bates No.
  2025431401/1406
  http://www.pmdocs.com/getallimg.asp?DOCID=2025431401/1406
ASIA IS NOW…
Dollisson J. Philip Morris 2nd Revised Forecast Presentation. June 1989 (est),
  Bates No. 2500101311/1323
  http://www.pmdocs.com/getallimg.asp?if=avpidx&DOCID=2500101311/13
  23
NATURALLY…
Kornegay H, Tobacco Institute, Speech to Tobacco and Allied Industries
  Division of the American Jewish Community on 11 December 1979, Bates
  No. TIMN0094652-4662,
  http://www.tobaccodocuments.org/view.cfm?docid=TIMN0094652/4662&
  source=SNAPTI&ShowImages=yes
DOCUMENT RETENTION POLICY…
Kremner C. US seeks facts on smoke conspiracy, *The Age*, 19 April 2002
  http://www.theage.com.au/articles/2002/04/18/1019020683796.html

40 MILLION PAGES
Balbach ED, Gasior RJ, Barbeau EM, Research paper: Tobacco industry
  documents: comparing the Minnesota Depository and internet access, *Tobacco
  Control* 2002, 11:68–72

TEXT
Glantz SA, Slade J, Bero LA, Hanauer P, Barnes DE (eds), *The Cigarette Papers*,
  University of California Press, 1996
Anon. Information: How to access tobacco industry documents. *Tobacco Control*
  2002, 11:i39

Part Five:
TAKING ACTION

22 Research

MAIN MAP

GYTS: Personal Communication, Wick Warren, CDC, 29 March, 2002

Fogarty: Personal Communication with Gerald Keusch, 28 May 2002

COMPARATIVE RESEARCH

Research expenditure, US National Institutes of Health, 2001, Research
Initiatives/Programs of Interest

http://www4.od.nih.gov/officeofbudget/FundingResearchAreas.htm,
downloaded 29 March 2002

DEATHS

Minino AM, Smith BL, Deaths: Preliminary data for 2000, *National Vital
Statistics Report*, Vol 49, No 12. Table 2, 9 October 2001, National Center for
Health Statistics, Centers for Disease Control and Prevention.

HOW MUCH RESEARCH?

Medline PubMed, US National Library of Medicine, 1 April 2002

TEXT

Baris et al, Research priorities for tobacco control in developing countries: A
regional approach to a global consultative process. *Tobacco Control* 9, 217–23,
2000.

Institute of Medicine (1998), *Control of CVD in Developing Countries*, National
Academy Press, Washington DC, USA

23 Tobacco Control Organisations

CLIPBOARD

Document: Cullman H. Philip Morris, Australia: smoking and health
strategy/Some recent developments in Australia. 1978 February. Bates MISC
2024978017/8049,
<http://www.tobaccodocuments.com/dispPage.cfm?SearchKey=administra
tion%20and%20threat&HideComment=YES&DisplayFormat=GIF&parentID
=39533> Text:
<http://www.tobacco.org/Documents/7802australia.html> Tobacco BBS.

TEXT

Brundtland GH, Director General Elect, The World Health Organization,
Geneva. Speech to the 51st World Health Assembly, 13 May 1998

24 Legislation: Smoke-free Areas

MAIN MAP

Corrao MA, Guidon GE, Sharma N, Shokoohi DF (eds), *Tobacco Control Country
Profiles*, American Cancer Society, Atlanta, GA, USA, 2000

Brownson RC, Hopkins DP, Wakefield MA, Effects of Smoking Restrictions in
the Workplace, *Annual Review of Public Health* 2002, 23:333–348

Public Support – Environics Research Group, "Citizens from Four Continents
Condemn Tobacco, Call for Tougher Regulation" 30 October 2001,
http://erg.environics.net/news/default.asp?aID=482

POLLUTED SPACES (BARCELONA)

Jané M, Nebot M, Rojano X, Artazcoz L, Sunyer J, Fernández E, Ceraso M,

Samet J, Hammond SK, Exposure to environmental tobacco smoke in public
places in Barcelona, Spain *Tobacco Control 2002*, 11: 83–84
http://www.tobaccocontrol.com/cgi/content/full/11/1/83

NO LOSS OF RESTAURANT AND BAR SALES

Before and After Smoke-free Laws First Quarter Taxable Sales Figures for
Restaurants & Bars, State of California 1992–1999, Source: California Dept.
of Health; California Board of Equalization, in: Repace J, Can Ventilation
Control Secondhand Smoke in the Hospitality Industry?, June 2000, Figure
3:34, http://www.repace.com

California Board of Equalization, 1997,1998,1999,2000,2001
http://www.boe.ca.gov/news/t1q99f.htm
http://www.boe.ca.gov/news/t11q0f.htm
http://www.boe.ca.gov/news/pdf/T11q01.pdf, etc

THE COST OF WORKPLACE SMOKING

Griffiths J, Grieves K, *Why Smoking in the Workplace Matters: An Employers Guide*,
WHO European Partnership Project to Reduce Tobacco Dependence,
2002:3

CLIPBOARD

Hieronimus J, Memorandum: Restrictions; bans, workplace smoking
restrictions; consumption.
Bates No.: 2023914280/4284.
http://www.pmdocs.com/getallimg.asp?if=avpidx&DOCID=2023914280/
4284. Philip Morris, USA, 22 October 1992

25 Legislation: Advertising Bans

MAIN MAP

Jha P, Chaloupka FJ, *Tobacco control in developing countries*, Oxford University
Press, 2000: 231–232

EFFECT OF AD BANS

Jha P, Chaloupka FJ, *Tobacco control in developing countries*, Oxford University
Press, 2000:224,233

CLIPBOARDS
ACTION PLAN...

RJ Reynolds, Tobacco Issues Strategy, 10 February 1989, Bates No. 507604596
IT IS FELT...

Miller L, Principles of measurement of visual standout in pack design, Report
No. RD 2039 Restricted, Group Research & Development Centre, British
American Tobacco Co. Ltd, May 23, 1986. Bates No. 102699347-102699500

TEXT

Jha P, Chaloupka FJ, *Tobacco Control in Developing Countries*, Oxford University
Press, 2000:229

Wakefield M, et al, The cigarette pack as image: new evidence from tobacco
industry documents, *Tobacco Control 2002*, 11(Suppl 1): i73–i80

Saffer H, Chaloupka FJ, The effect of advertising on tobacco consumption,
Journal of Health Economics 2000; 19: 1117–37

26 Legislation: Health Warnings

MAIN MAP

Corrao MA, Guidon GE, Sharma N, Shokoohi DF (eds), *Tobacco Control Country
Profiles*, American Cancer Society, Atlanta, GA, USA, 2000.

World Health Organization, Tobacco Free Initiative, Legislative Measures
adopted by WHO Member & Associated States, 24 May 2000, (unpublished)

PUBLIC SUPPORT

Environics Research Group. Citizens from Four Continents Condemn Tobacco, Call for Tougher Regulation. 30 October 2001, http://erg.environics.net/news/default.asp?aID=482

HEALTH WARNINGS IN CANADA

Canadian Cancer Society, Press Release, 9 January 2002
http://www.ontario.cancer.ca/siteboth/english/cigarette_package_warnings.asp

CLIPBOARD

IF THEY REJECT YOUR PACK…

Ludo Cremers, Divisional vice president of marketing, Brown and Williamson, a division of BAT, 2002, http://online.wsj.com/article/0,,BT_CO_20020506_003393,00.html

TEXT

Quote: ASH SCOTLAND. Policy Paper on Regulation and Control of Tobacco Products: Packaging/Labelling, downloaded 11 April 2002 http://www.ashscotland.org.uk/issues/tob_reg09.html

Tobacco Warning Labels and Packaging Fact Sheet, prepared for 11th World Conference on Tobacco or Health, 2000

27 Health Education

MAIN MAP AND QUIT & WIN CAMPAIGN

Personal communication, Patrick Sandstrom, Eeva Riitta Vartiainen, Quit & Win Campaign, Finland, April 2002

CLIPBOARDS

PUBLIC STATEMENT

Philip Morris billboard, January 1990
http://tobaccodocuments.org/landman/137755.html

PRIVATE STATEMENT

Discussion Paper. 29 January 1991. Site: Tobacco Institute document site http://www.tobaccoinstitute.com/

Bates No. TIMN0164422/4424 (and also other Bates No. TIFL0526381/6383), http://www.tobaccoinstitute.com/getallimg.asp?DOCID=TIMN0164422/4424

TEXT

Environics Research Group, 2001
http://erg.environics.net/news/default.asp?aid=482

28 Quitting

MAIN MAP

Algeria, 2000, *11th World Conference on Tobacco OR Health: Abstracts Vol.2* (Chicago, IL)
Austria, 2000, *Wiener Medizinische Wochenschrift*, 150(6), 109–114
Bahamas, 1992, *Tobacco or Health: Status in the Americas*, Washington, D.C.
Chile, 2000, *Pan American Journal of Public Health*, 7(2), 79–87
China, 2001, *Tobacco Control*, 10(2), 170–174
Côte d'Ivoire, 1981, Poumon-Coeur, 37, 87–94
Cyprus, *Research Papers and Reports: Series II*, Report no. 19, ISBN 9963-34-344-9
Czech Republic, 2000, *Casopis Lekaru Ceskych*, 139(5), 143–147
Denmark, 1992, *International Journal of Epidemiology*, 21(5), 862–871
Dominican Republic, 1993, *Bulletin of PAHO*, 27(4), 370–381
Ecuador, 1992, *Tobacco or Health: Status in the Americas*, Washington, D.C.
Egypt, 1982, Provided to the ACS; from the first cycle of *The Health Interview Survey of Egypt*
Finland, 1998, Provided to the ACS; data from *Health Behavior among Finnish Adult Population*, spring 1998
France, 2000, *International Journal of Tuberculosis and Lung Disease*, 4(8), 698–704
Germany, 1999, Jahrbuch Sucht
Ghana, a pamphlet sent to ACS by the Health and Humanitarian Environment Society
Honduras, 1992, *Tobacco or Health: Status in the Americas*, Washington, D.C.

Iran (Islamic Republic of), 2000, *11th World Conference on Tobacco OR Health: Abstracts Vol. 2* (Chicago, IL)
Israel, 2000, *The Israeli Medical Journal*, 2(5), 351–355
Kuwait, 2000, *Bulletin of the World Health Organization*, 78(11), 1306–1315
Malawi, 1996, *Tropical Doctor*, 26(3),139
Mexico, 1998, Unpublished Data
Peru, 1992, PAHO publication
Russian Federation, 2000, *11th World Conference on Tobacco OR Health: Abstracts Vol. 2* (Chicago, IL)
Saudi Arabia, 2001, *National Study on Coronary Artery Risk Factors*, 1996–2001
South Africa, 2000, *11th World Conference on Tobacco OR Health: Abstracts Vol. 2* (Chicago, IL)
Sudan, 2000, *11th World Conference on Tobacco OR Health: Abstracts Vol. 2* (Chicago, IL)
Sweden, 2001, *Tobacco Control*, 10, 258–266
Thailand, 1993, Thailand's Situation. Online: www.ash.or.th/situation/women.htm
Tonga, 1994, *Tobacco Control*, 3, 41–45
Trinidad and Tobago, 1992, *Tobacco or Health: Status in the Americas*, Washington DC
Turkey, 1998, *Lung Cancer*, 21, 127–132
Tuvalu, 1986, *Bulletin of the World Health Organization*, 64(3), 447–456, data was provided to the ACS
USA, 2000, *11th World Conference on Tobacco OR Health: Abstracts Vol. 2* (Chicago, IL)
Uruguay, 2000, *11th World Conference on Tobacco OR Health: Abstracts Vol. 2* (Chicago, IL)
Venezuela, 1994, provided to the ACS via fax
Zambia, pre-publication results of a survey in Mutendere, a suburb of Lusaka. Mulenga M, Haworth A, Mwanza P

SYMBOL

NRT OTC: Personal communication, World Self-Medication Industry, April 2002

EFFECTS OF STARTING AND QUITTING SMOKING ON DEATHS

Peto R, Lopez AD, The future worldwide health effects of current smoking patterns, in: Koop EC, Pearson CE, Schwarz MR, eds, *Critical Issues in Global Health*, New York, Jossey-Bass, 2001:154–161

EFFECT OF SMOKING RESTRICTIONS AT HOME AND AT WORK

Farkas AJ, Gilpin EA, Distefan JM, Pierce JP, The effects of household and workplace smoking restrictions on quitting behaviours, *Tobacco Control 1999*, 8:261–265, Autumn

IMPACT OF INTERVENTIONS

Ross H, Chaloupka FJ, Jha P, Effectiveness of control policies for tobacco initiation and cessation, ITEN Working Paper Series, www.tobaccoevidence.net, November 2001

TEXT

Clive Bates quote, personal communication, June 2002

29 Price Policy

MAIN MAP AND SYMBOL

Jha P, Chaloupka FJ, *Tobacco Control in Developing Countries*, Oxford University Press, 2000. Table 10.1 and Table 17.4:239–240,421

TAX DOWN BUT PRICES UP

Sinful Tax, *New York Times*, 18 March 2002 *The Tax Burden on Tobacco*, Historical Compilation, Volume 35, 2000

SMOKING GOES DOWN AS PRICES GO UP

Abedian I, van der Merw R, Wilkins N, Jha P, *The Economics of Tobacco Control: Towards an optimal policy mix*, Applied Fiscal Research Centre, University of Cape Town, South Africa, 1998. Figure 1, Page 186. Source Townsend J, 1998

GOVERNMENT INCOME FROM TOBACCO

Jha P, Chaloupka FJ, *Tobacco Control in Developing Countries*, Oxford University Press, 2000, Table 10.2:255

CLIPBOARD

Smoking and Health Initiatives, Philip Morris International, 1985, Bates number 202326832949

TEXT

Adam Smith, *An Inquiry into the Nature and Causes of the Wealth of Nations* 1776

Jha P, Chaloupka FJ, *Tobacco Control in Developing Countries*, Oxford University Press, 2000, Table 10.1 and Table 17.4: 239–240, 421

30 Litigation

MAIN MAP & SMUGGLING LITIGATION

Personal communication with Professor Richard Daynard, Professor of Law, Northeastern University, USA, 2002

BAT FACED 4,419

British American Tobacco. Annual Review and Summary Financial Statement 2001, US litigation:38

CLIPBOARD

Edwards J. Report from Philip Morris Counsel to Philip Morris Counsel Regarding Meeting on Addiction. 6 November 1986. Bates No.: 2025005346/5367,
http://www.tobaccodocuments.org/view.cfm?docid=25156&source=B LILEY&ShowImages=yes

TEXT

Daynard RA, Bates C, Francey N, Tobacco litigation worldwide, *British Medical Journal*, 8 January 2000, 320: 111–113

Walburn RB, The prospects for globalizing tobacco litigation, WHO's International Conference on Global Tobacco Control Law: *Towards a WHO Framework Convention on Tobacco Control*, New Delhi, India, 7 January 2000

Blanke DD, *Towards Health with Justice: Litigation and public inquiries as tools for tobacco control*, World Health Organization (WHO), 18 March 2002
http://tobacco.who.int/repository/stp69/final_jordan_report.pdf ID: 88634

31 Projections by Industry

MAIN MAP

ERC, *The World Cigarette Market: The 1999 Survey*, ERC Group plc, 2000

TEXT

World Health Organization, Geneva, press release, WHO/2:16.1.1986

32 Future

TIMELINE

Mackay J, *Lessons from the Conference: The Next 25 years*, 10th World Conference on Tobacco or Health. Beijing, China, 24–28 August 1997

Future Scenarios Plenary, *Tobacco Control 2015: Where, Why and With What Outcomes?* 11th World Conference on Tobacco or Health, Chicago Illinois, 6–11 August 2000

Murray CJL, Lopez AD, *The Global Burden of Disease*, World Health Organization, Harvard School of Public Health, World Bank, 1996:38

Peto R and Lopez AD, personal communication 12 April 2002

TEXT

Lewin L, *Phantastica: Narcotic and Stimulating Drugs. Their Use and Abuse*, 1924, translated by PHA Wirth, 1931

Lopez AD, personal communication 12 April 2002

Part Six:
WORLD TABLES

Table A The Demographics of Tobacco

1. POPULATION
http://www.who.int/whr/2001/main/en/annex/annex1.htm
2. ADULT SMOKING
see sources for map 3: Main Map
3. YOUTH SMOKING
see sources for map 5: Maps
4. YOUTH EXPOSED TO PASSIVE SMOKING AT HOME
see sources for map 8: Children exposed to passive smoking at home.
5. CIGARETTE CONSUMPTION
see sources for map 6: Main Map
6. QUITTING
see sources for map 28: Main Map

Table B The Business of Tobacco

1. GROWING TOBACCO
columns 1 & 2: see sources for Map 12: Main Map
column 3: see sources for Map 12: Leading producers of Tobacco Leaves
2. TOBACCO TRADE
columns 1 & 2: see sources for Map 15, Main Map
columns 3 & 4: see sources for Map 15, Tobacco Leaves inset
3. MANUFACTURING TOBACCO
column 1: see sources for Map 13: Main Map
column 2: USDA, Economic Research Service, Tobacco Statistics (94102) Table 167, World Cigarette Production, Selected Countries, 1960–1995, USDA website accessed January 2002,
http://www.ers.usda.gov/data/sdp/view.asp?f=specialty/94012/
4. COSTS
columns 1 & 2: see sources for Map 11, Main Map
columns 3 & 4: see sources for Map 11, A Hard Day's Smoke
5. TAX
column 1: see sources for Map 29, Main Map
column 2: see sources for Map 29, Government income from Tobacco
6. TOBACCO INDUSTRY DOCUMENTS
see sources for Map 21: Main Map

Glossary

Bates C, McNeill A, Jarvis M, Gray M, The future of tobacco product regulation and labelling in Europe: implications for the forthcoming European Union directive, *Tobacco Control 1999*, 8: 225–235

Glantz S, *Model Tobacco Education Legislation*, Version 6; February 3, 1999

Jha P, Chaloupka FJ, *Tobacco Control in Developing Countries*, Oxford University Press, 2000: 464–469

World Health Organization, *Guidelines for controlling and monitoring the tobacco epidemic*, WHO, Geneva, 1998: 123–125

Tobacco or Health: A Global Status Report, WHO, Geneva, 1997

USEFUL CONTACTS

WHO Tobacco Free Initiative

WHO Headquarters
  http://tobacco.who.int/
AFRO
  http://www.whoafr.org/tfi/index.html
EMRO
  http://www.emro.who.int/tfi/tfi.htm
EURO
  http://www.who.dk/eprise/main/WHO/Progs/TOB/Home
PAHO
  http://www.paho.org/
SEARO
  http://w3.whosea.org/techinfo/index.htm
WPRO
  http://www.wpro.who.int/themes_focuses/theme2/special/tobacco.asp

International Organisations

Tobacco Documents Online (TDO, Smokescreen)
  http://www.tobaccodocuments.org
Framework Convention Alliance (FCA) http://www.fctc.org/
Global Partnerships for Tobacco Control
  http://www.essentialaction.org/tobacco/
GLOBALink, UICC International Union Against Cancer
  http://www.globalink.org/
Hamman's research site (Steve Hamann)
  http://hamann.globalink.org/ (or)
http://www.thai.net/tobaccocontrol/
International Agency on Tobacco and Health (IATH)
  email: admin@iath.org
International Network of Women Against Tobacco (INWAT)
  http://www.inwat.org/
International Network Towards Smoke-Free Hospitals (INTSH)
  http://intsh.globalink.org/
International Non Governmental Coalition Against Tobacco
  (INGCAT)
  http://www.ingcat.org/
International Society for the Prevention of Tobacco Induced Diseases
  (PTID)
  http://www.ptid.org/
International Tobacco Evidence Network (ITEN)
  http://www.tobaccoevidence.net/
Legacy Foundation, tobacco document site
  http://legacy.library.ucsf.edu/cgi/b/bib/bib-idx?g=tob
Network for Accountability of Tobacco Transnationals (NATT)
  www.infact.org
Quit&Win
  http://www.quitandwin.org
Repace's site, especially on passive smoking (Jim Repace)
  http://www.repace.com/

Smokescreen Action Network (Michael Tacelosky)
  http://www.smokescreen.org
Society for Research on Nicotine and Tobacco (SRNT)
  http://www.srnt.org/
Tobacco BBS (Gene Borio)
  http://www.tobacco.org
Tobacco Control journal
  http://www.tobaccocontrol.com
Tobacco Control Resource Center/Tobacco Products Liability Project
  (TCRC/TPLP)
  http://tobacco.neu.edu/
Tobacco Control Resource Centre (TCRC), BMA, UK
  http://www.tobacco-control.org/
Tobacco Control Supersite (Simon Chapman)
  http://www.health.usyd.edu.au/tobacco/
Tobaccopedia
  http://TobaccoPedia.org
Treatobacco Database & Educational Resource for Treatment of
  Tobacco Dependence
  http://www.treatobacco.net/
12th World Conference on Tobacco or Health, Helsinki, 3–8 August
  2003
  http://www.wctoh2003.org

Regional Organisations

European Medical Association on Smoking and Health (EMASH)
  http://emash.globalink.org/
European Network for Smoke-free Hospitals (ENSH)
  http://ensh.free.fr/
European Network for Smoking Prevention (ENSP)
  http://www.ensp.org
European Network of Young People and Tobacco
  http://www.ktl.fi/enypat/
European Network of Quitlines
  http://www.quitlines-conference.com/
Southeast Asian Tobacco Control Alliance
  http://www.tobaccofreeasia.net/
Tobacco Free Forum, South Asia Association for Regional
  Cooperation
  http://wbb.globalink.org

These web and email addresses were accurate in mid-2002. There
are, in addition, many other organisations, wholly or partly working
on tobacco issues, too numerous to include here. These can be
contacted through INGCAT (the International Non Governmental
Coalition Against Tobacco) or WHO. If any would like to be included
in future editions, or on a website, please contact the authors.

In addition, we were unable to include any national and sub-
national organisations.

INDEX